VEGAN

BODYBUILDING

Cookbook for men

Build muscle, become lean, and maintain your health with these 100 vegan recipes for fitness enthusiasts, athletes, and sports fans.

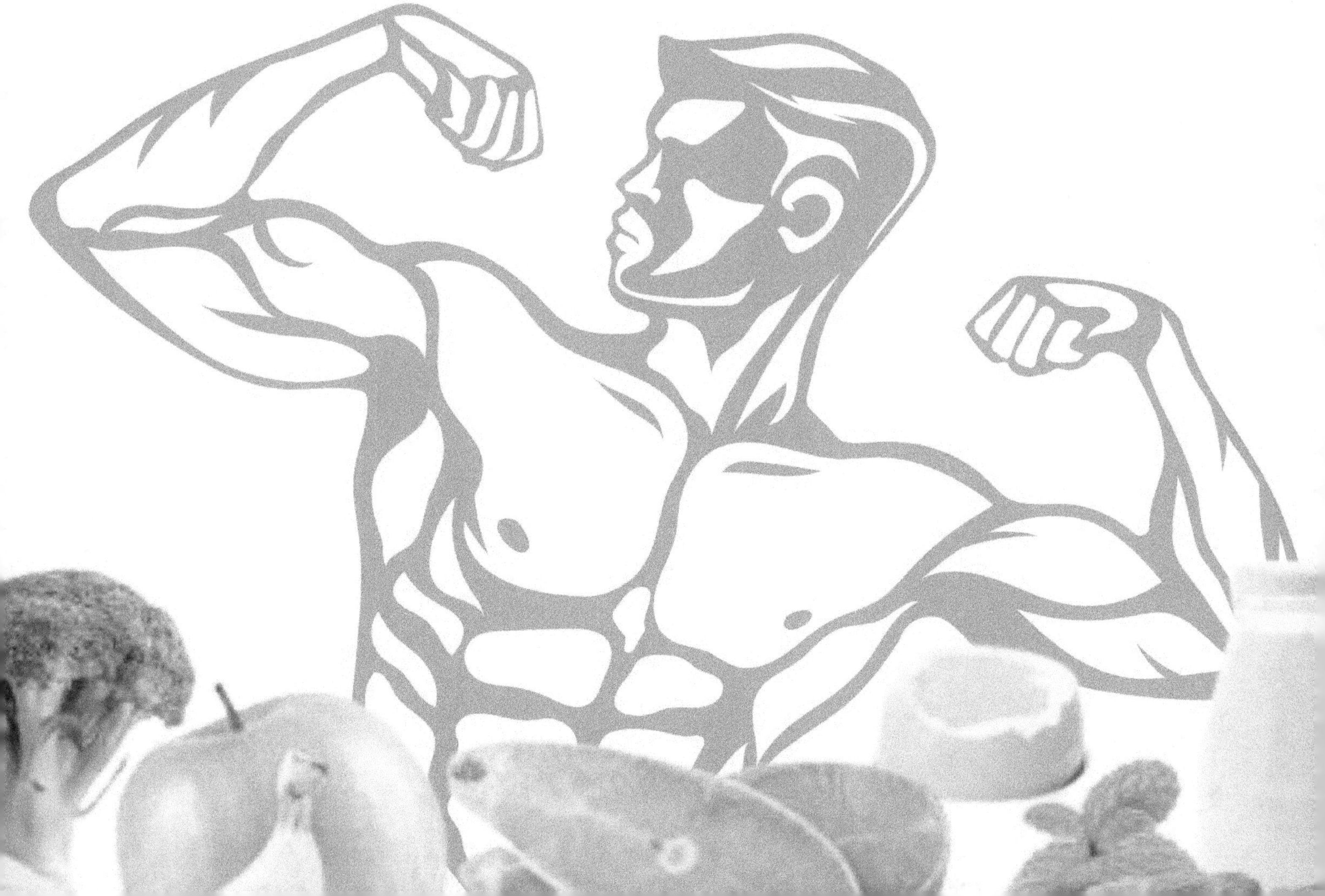

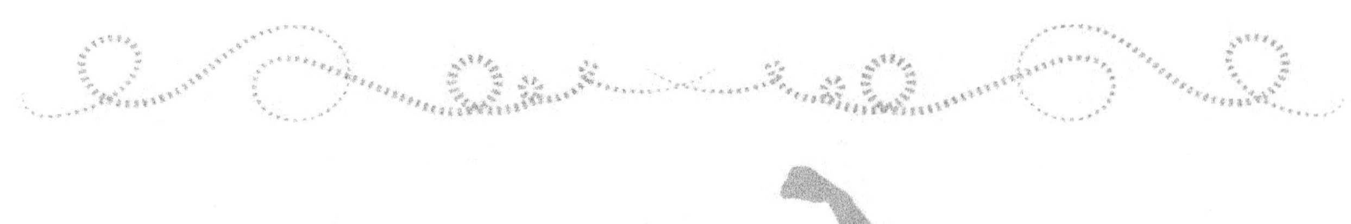

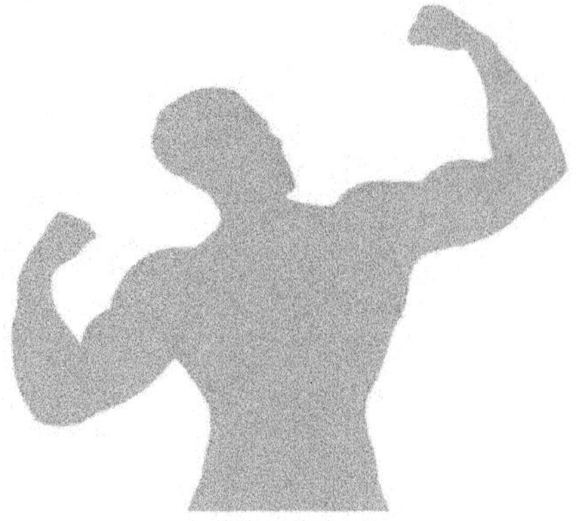

Copyright © 2024 Sarah William

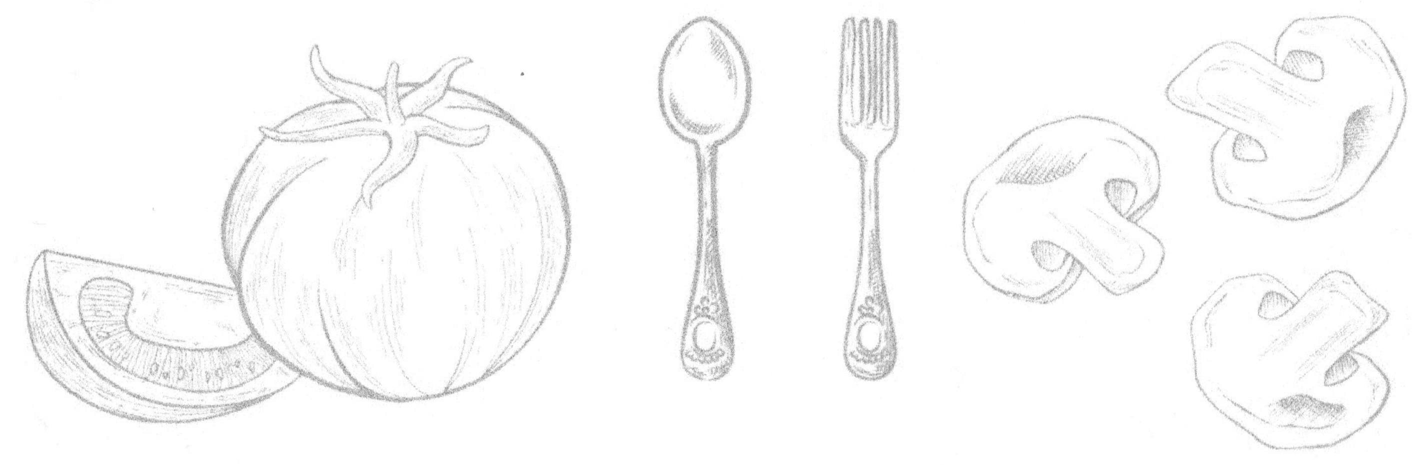

TABLE OF CONTENTS

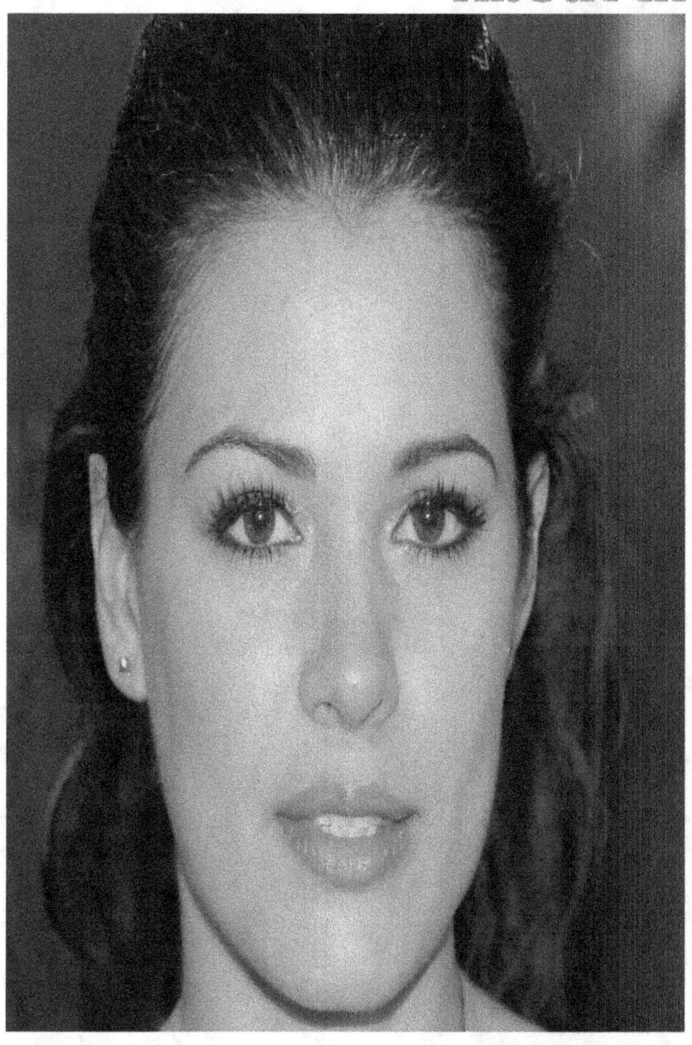

Sarah William is a fervent supporter of holistic health, exercise, and plant-based diets. Sarah, who has a degree in nutrition and a strong passion for food, has made it her mission to educate others about the transforming potential of veganism.

Sarah has worked with clients from many walks of life, assisting them on their path to optimum health and vitality as a certified personal trainer and health coach. Her strategy is based on empathy, knowledge, and empowerment, enabling people to take charge of their health and adopt more sustainable lifestyles.

Sarah's desire to match her food choices with her ethical principles led her to become a vegan more than ten years ago. What began as a personal journey towards sustainability and health quickly became a lifetime passion and goal to encourage others to adopt a plant-based diet.

Apart from her occupation as a health and fitness specialist, Sarah enjoys cooking and creating new recipes. She shares her passion for tasty, wholesome, and cruelty-free food with a worldwide audience via her blog, social media accounts, and now her Vegan Bodybuilding Cookbook.

Sarah enjoys hiking in the outdoors, doing yoga, or curling up with a good book and a cup of herbal tea when she's not in the kitchen trying out new recipes or working out at the gym.

Sarah thinks that we may reach our greatest potential and lead vibrant, meaningful lives by providing our bodies with healthful, plant-based meals and our brains with good ideas and aspirations.

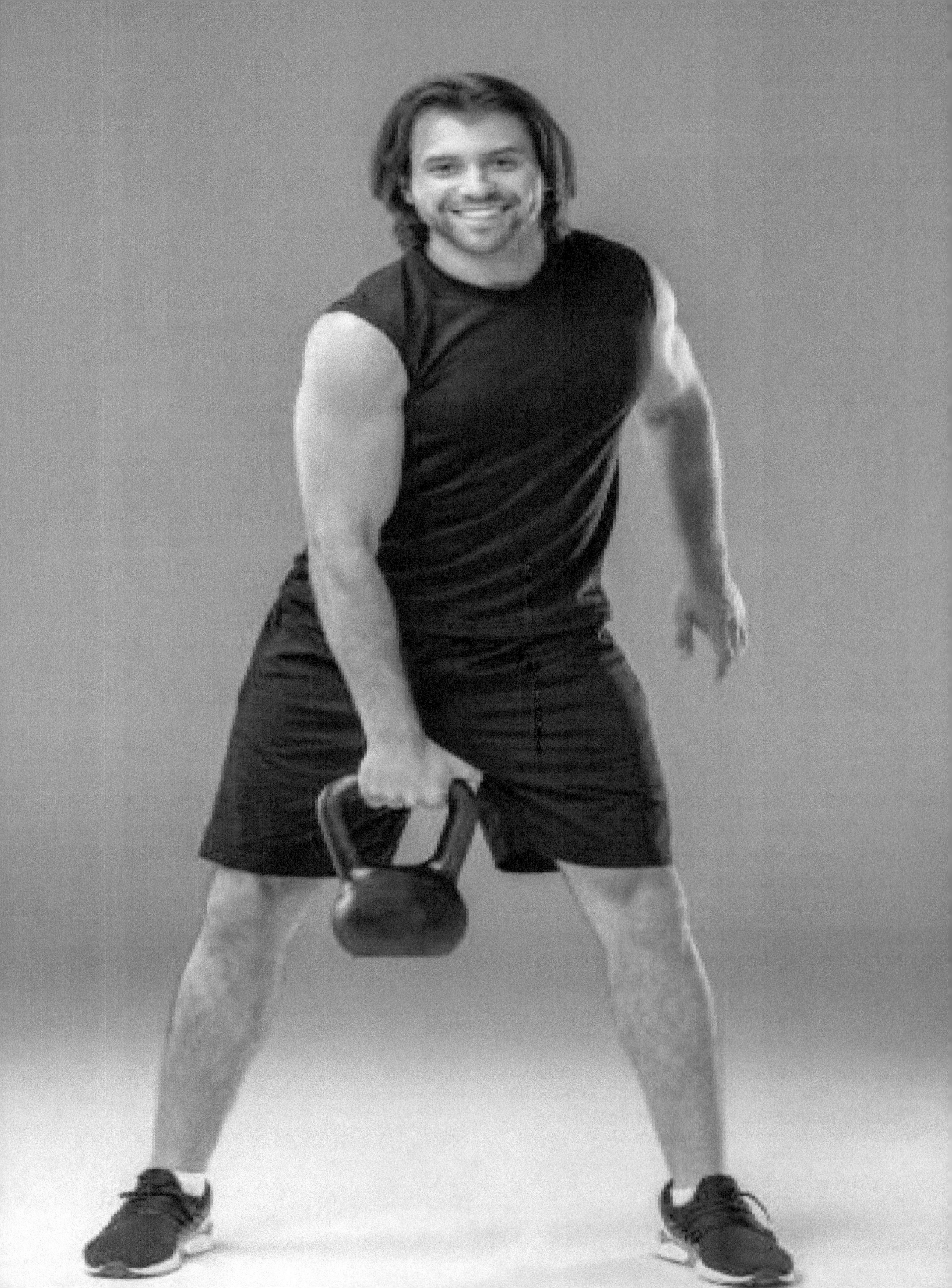

Introduction

Welcome to the world of vegan bodybuilding, a powerful way of life where compassion, vigor, and strength join together. As an experienced athlete and committed vegan, I've started a life-changing adventure that has changed not only my physical appearance but also my perspective on well-being, health, and the interdependence of all living things.

Being a competitive athlete in my early years sparked my enthusiasm for nutrition and fitness. I was a competitive player who pushed my body to the limit, but I quickly learned that genuine strength is more than simply physical ability. It calls for an all-encompassing strategy that takes care of the body, mind, and soul.

Making the switch to a vegan diet was a turning point in my development as an athlete. I was first faced with doubt and suspicion, but I quickly learned that there was a wealth of plant-based meals that may enhance performance, hasten recovery, and fuel my workouts. The days of just eating animal products were over. I now embraced a vibrant variety of fruits, vegetables, legumes, and grains that gave me all the nutrients I needed to be healthy.

I developed my cooking abilities by trial and error, creating delectable and nourishing meals that aided in the achievement of my fitness objectives. Every dish turned into a demonstration of the plant-based miracle that is vegan cooking, highlighting its limitless potential. I felt content with every bite of whatever I ate, from protein-rich smoothie bowls to filling grain bowls and decadent sweets, since I was feeding my body by my moral principles.

But my quest was much more than simply getting a toned body or packing on muscle; it was about getting my health and energy back from the inside out. I saw a significant shift in my body that went far beyond the gym when I adopted a plant-based diet. In addition to feeling lighter, I also felt more energized and a part of the world. My days of feeling lethargic and having stomach problems were over.

Instead, I was filled with renewed energy and an overall feeling of well-being that came from the inside out.

Now that I'm an authority on health and well-being, I'm excited to impart my wisdom to you in my Vegan Bodybuilding Cookbook for Men. This book is your road map to maximizing the benefits of plant-based nutrition, regardless of your level of experience with fitness, athletic ability, or simple interest in sports and health.

There are one hundred delectable recipes that will help you nourish your body, gain muscle, and maintain an active lifestyle. Every meal, from filling lunches to delicious evenings and everything in between, is carefully prepared to maximize taste and nutritional value. This cookbook includes recipes that will help you achieve your goals of losing weight, recovering after exercise, and enjoying tasty, healthful cuisine.

Come along with me on this incredible quest for vegan bodybuilding prowess. Honoring our bodies, our world, and the creatures we share it with, we'll reinvent what it means to be strong, vibrant, and unstoppable together.

Cheers to your well-being, tenacity, and boundless possibilities.

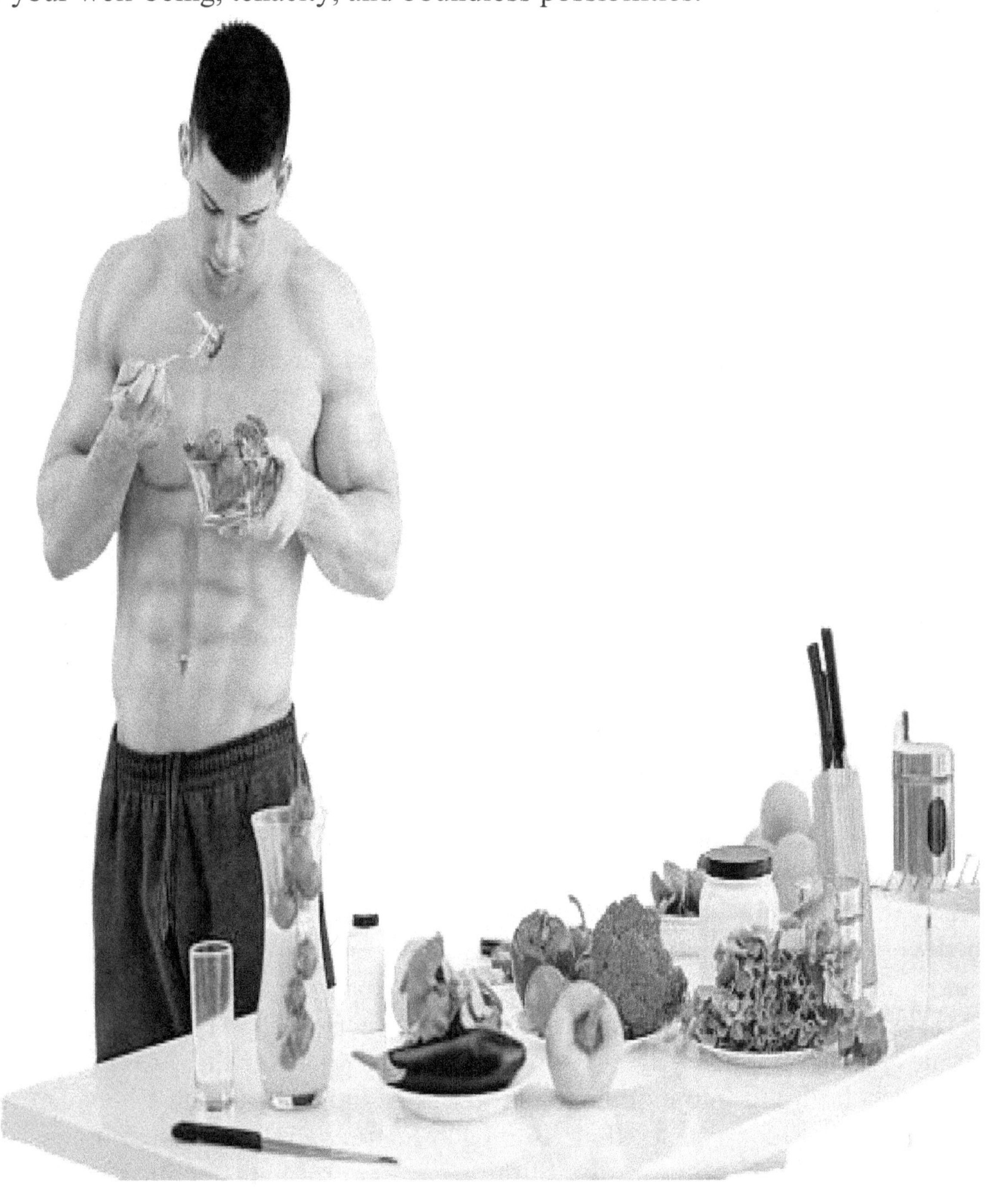

Understanding Vegan Bodybuilding

Allow me to take you back to the start of my vegan bodybuilding career when it seemed unimaginable that one could gain muscle on a plant-based diet. Like most of you, I had my doubts. Without the conventional mainstays of meat, eggs, and dairy, how could I ever hope to reach my fitness goals?

However, when I learned more about the vegan diet, I was able to dispel the myths and false beliefs that had influenced my perception. I discovered that in addition to being high in protein, plant-based diets are also a great source of important vitamins, minerals, and antioxidants that are critical for healthy overall development, recuperation, and muscular building.

Through my personal experiences, I learned that being a vegan bodybuilder is about adopting a varied, nutrient-dense diet that feeds the body from the inside out, rather than merely replacing animal goods with plant-based alternatives. It's about coming up with inventive methods to acquire the protein you need from complete foods like lentils, beans, tofu, and tempeh. To maximize your nutritional intake and support your workout program, you should also include a rainbow of fruits and vegetables.

The relationship between my food choices and my performance in the gym, however, was maybe the most significant insight I discovered along the way. My energy levels, endurance, and recovery times all improved when I made the switch to a plant-based diet. I no longer regarded hefty, animal-based meals to be a burden; instead, I felt lighter, more flexible, and more robust than before.

As I developed my vegan bodybuilding strategy further, I also saw how my nutritional decisions affected other aspects of my life. By choosing plant-based protein sources, I was improving not only my health but also the health of animals throughout the globe and my environmental impact. It was a profound insight that gave my trip more depth and meaning, stoking my enthusiasm for veganism and encouraging others to follow me on this life-changing adventure.

I thus encourage everyone who aspires to be a vegan bodybuilder to approach this adventure with bravery and an open mind. Put your faith in plants' ability to improve your health, shape your body, and fuel your workouts. And never forget, one plant-based meal at a time, you're not only growing muscle, you're creating a better planet.

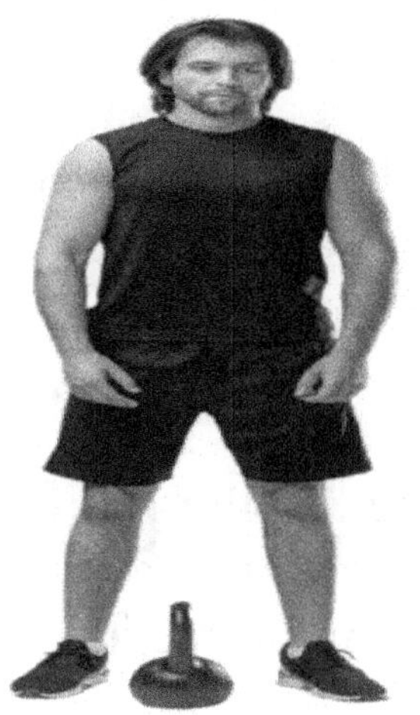

The conventional bodybuilding narrative often centers on animal-based protein sources like eggs, meat, and chicken. But as a vegan bodybuilder, I've learned to value the many advantages a plant-based diet provides for reaching peak performance, building muscle, and maintaining general health.

The richness of nutrients in plant-based diets is one of the biggest benefits of veganism for bodybuilders. Plant-based sources are abundant in protein, vital amino acids, vitamins, minerals, and antioxidants, despite popular belief to the contrary. These nutrients are critical for promoting muscle development, mending tissue damage, and improving recuperation.

Furthermore, compared to animal products, plant-based diets are often lower in cholesterol and saturated fats, making them a heart-healthy choice for athletes who are worried about their general and cardiovascular health. Bodybuilders who follow a vegan diet may preserve their lean muscle mass and lower their chance of developing chronic illnesses like diabetes, heart disease, and certain types of cancer by opting for whole, minimally processed plant foods.

Moreover, a plant-based diet provides better digestion advantages, supporting gut health and nutrient absorption—an essential component for athletes looking to maximize their recuperation and performance. Vegan bodybuilders may promote healthy microbiota, ease digestive pain, and guarantee optimal nutrition utilization for maximal gains by emphasizing fiber-rich fruits, vegetables, whole grains, and legumes.

However, the strongest argument in favor of veganism for bodybuilding may come from ethical and environmental factors as well as physical benefits. Vegan bodybuilders use plant-based protein sources instead of animal products to ensure that their diets reflect their commitment to environmental stewardship, sustainability, and compassion. They provide their bodies with healthful, plant-based nourishment while simultaneously lowering the need for factory farming, minimizing animal suffering, and lessening the negative environmental effects of animal agriculture.

To sum up, there are many advantages to veganism for bodybuilders beyond just improved physical health. These advantages include ethical, environmental, and even spiritual aspects. Vegan bodybuilders may attain their fitness objectives and advance sustainability, compassion, and well-being for themselves, the environment, and future generations by adopting a plant-based diet. This win-win-win situation shows how plant-based nutrition may revolutionize bodybuilding and other industries.

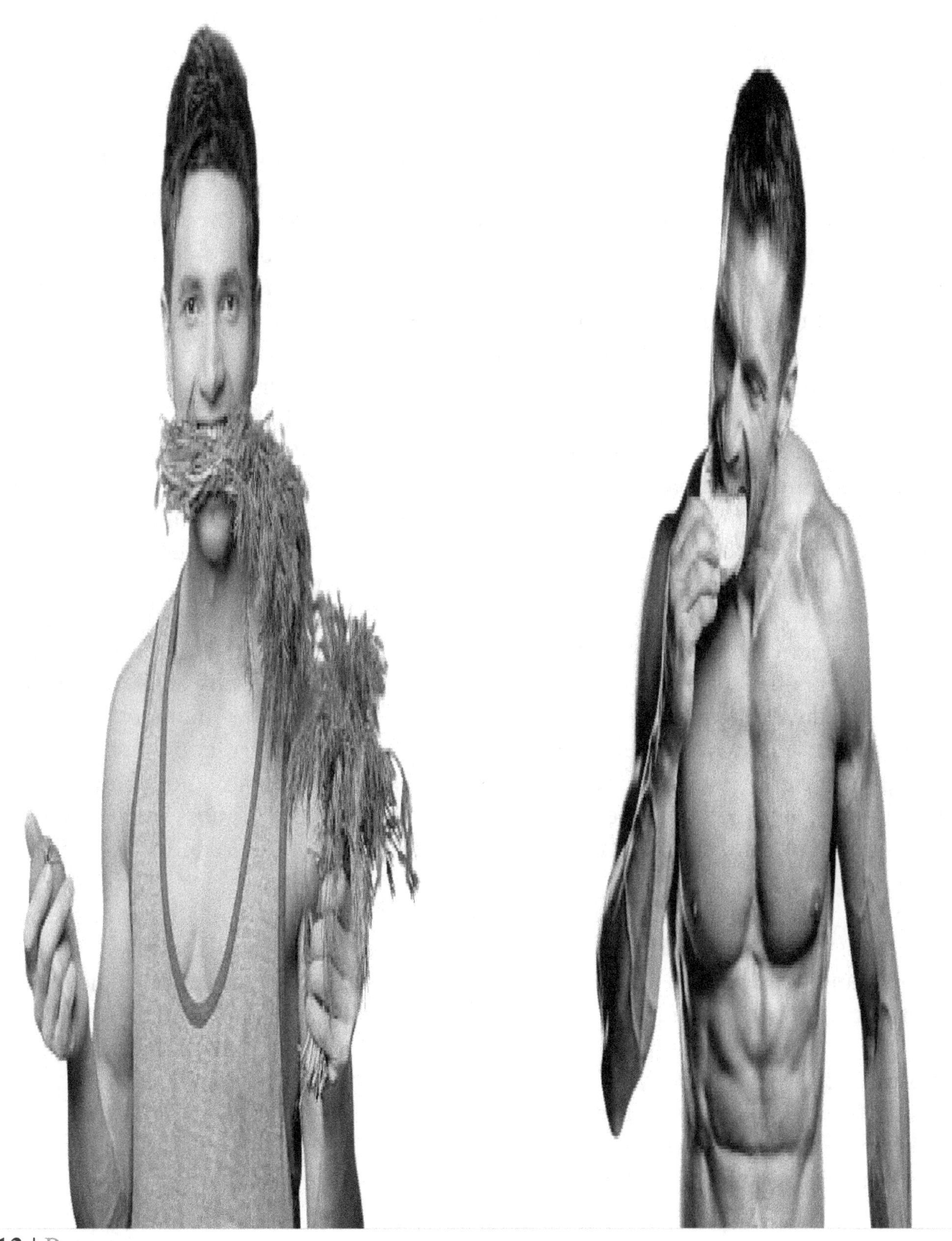

The conventional bodybuilding narrative often centers on animal-based protein sources like eggs, meat, and chicken. But as a vegan bodybuilder, I've learned to value the many advantages a plant-based diet provides for reaching peak performance, building muscle, and maintaining general health.

The richness of nutrients in plant-based diets is one of the biggest benefits of veganism for bodybuilders. Plant-based sources are abundant in protein, vital amino acids, vitamins, minerals, and antioxidants, despite popular belief to the contrary. These nutrients are critical for promoting muscle development, mending tissue damage, and improving recuperation.

Furthermore, compared to animal products, plant-based diets are often lower in cholesterol and saturated fats, making them a heart-healthy choice for athletes who are worried about their general and cardiovascular health. Bodybuilders who follow a vegan diet may preserve their lean muscle mass and lower their chance of developing chronic illnesses like diabetes, heart disease, and certain types of cancer by opting for whole, minimally processed plant foods.

Moreover, a plant-based diet provides better digestion advantages, supporting gut health and nutrient absorption—an essential component for athletes looking to maximize their recuperation and performance. Vegan bodybuilders may promote healthy microbiota, ease digestive pain, and guarantee optimal nutrition utilization for maximal gains by emphasizing fiber-rich fruits, vegetables, whole grains, and legumes.

However, the strongest argument in favor of veganism for bodybuilding may come from ethical and environmental factors as well as physical benefits. Vegan bodybuilders use plant-based protein sources instead of animal products to ensure that their diets reflect their commitment to environmental stewardship, sustainability, and compassion. They provide their bodies with healthful, plant-based nourishment while simultaneously lowering the need for factory farming, minimizing animal suffering, and lessening the negative environmental effects of animal agriculture.

To sum up, there are many advantages to veganism for bodybuilders beyond just improved physical health. These advantages include ethical, environmental, and even spiritual aspects. Vegan bodybuilders may attain their fitness objectives and advance sustainability, compassion, and well-being for themselves, the environment, and future generations by adopting a plant-based diet. This win-win-win situation shows how plant-based nutrition may revolutionize bodybuilding and other industries.

The process of building muscle is intricate and depends on the cooperative effects of many nutrients to promote protein synthesis, aid in tissue restoration, and enhance recuperation. While protein is often the main topic of conversation when it comes to muscle development, several other essential nutrients are just as important for fostering muscle growth and improving overall athletic performance.

First and foremost, protein is necessary to promote muscle protein synthesis and serves as the building block of muscle tissue. As the building blocks of new muscle tissue and essential for the repair and rebuilding of muscle fibers destroyed during exercise, amino acids are the individual components of protein. Plant-based sources of protein that vegan bodybuilders may consume in sufficient amounts include beans, lentils, tofu, tempeh, quinoa, and seitan.

Carbohydrates, in addition to protein, are essential for promoting muscle development because they provide the energy required for activity and the replenishment of glycogen reserves afterward. During high-intensity activity, the body uses carbohydrates as its main fuel source; thus, consuming too few carbohydrates may cause weariness, a decline in performance, and difficulties in recovery. Excellent sources of complex carbohydrates that maintain energy levels and promote peak athletic performance include whole grains, fruits, vegetables, and legumes.

Another vital component for building muscle is healthy fats, which also help with food absorption, hormone synthesis, and focused energy generation. Particularly, omega-3 and omega-6 fatty acids are crucial for joint health, inflammation control, and general well-being. A vegan bodybuilder may include foods high in healthy fats, like as nuts, seeds, avocados, and plant oils, in their diet to aid in muscle building and recuperation.

Vitamins and minerals are examples of micronutrients that are essential for both general health and muscular development. In addition to vitamins D and K, which are crucial for calcium metabolism and bone remodeling, calcium, magnesium, and phosphorus are necessary for healthy bones and muscular contraction. Antioxidants that promote recovery and guard against oxidative damage brought on by exercise include vitamin C, vitamin E, and selenium.

Beyond protein, other important nutrients for muscle building include lipids, carbs, vitamins, and minerals. Plant-based protein, carbs, and healthy fats are abundant in plant-based diets, which vegan bodybuilders prioritize to support muscle building, maximize performance, and promote overall health and well-being. Vegan athletes may thrive on a plant-based diet and meet their fitness objectives by paying close attention to their nutritional demands and using appropriate fuelling tactics.

Kitchen Essentials for Vegan Bodybuilders

Being a vegan bodybuilder means having to cook with a well-stocked kitchen full of supplies, utensils, and appliances in order to create wholesome and tasty meals. With the correct tools and pantry essentials on hand, you can create tasty meals that stimulate muscle building and fuel your exercises, whether you're making a substantial grain bowl or a protein-packed smoothie.

A well-stocked pantry is a must for vegan bodybuilders, to begin with. This contains a range of whole grains, including barley, quinoa, brown rice, and oats, which provide complex carbs for long-lasting energy and serve as a wholesome foundation for meals. Additionally helpful, legumes such as beans, lentils, and chickpeas provide fiber, plant-based protein, and vital elements for the development and repair of muscles.

Healthy fats, protein, and micronutrients are provided by a variety of nuts, seeds, and nut butter in addition to grains and legumes, supporting general health and well-being. Nuts like almonds, walnuts, chia seeds, and flaxseeds are great ways to enhance the taste, texture, and nutritional content of meals and snacks.

A high-speed blender is an essential piece of kitchen equipment for vegan bodybuilders. Smooth and silky textures may be achieved by swiftly and effectively breaking down components in a powerful blender, whether you're mixing up protein-rich smoothies, creamy sauces, or nutrient-dense soups. In order to handle difficult items like frozen fruits and veggies, look for a blender with robust blades and numerous speed settings.

Cooking substantial foods like spaghetti, stews, and stir-fries also needs a good collection of pots and pans. Choose cookware made of stainless steel or non-stick that can tolerate high heat and provide uniform cooking so you can consistently get excellent results. For safe and effective food preparation, it's also critical to invest in high-quality kitchen knives and cutting boards, which make it simple to chop, slice, and dice items.

Last, but not least, remember to pack your nutrient-dense masterpieces in meal prep containers and carry along portable snacks for on-the-go energy. Reusable water bottles and shaker cups are great for keeping hydrated and quickly preparing protein shakes, while glass or BPA-free plastic containers are great for holding batch-cooked meals and pre-portioned snacks.

Having these basics in your kitchen will make it easier for you to make wholesome, tasty meals that will help you achieve your vegan bodybuilding objectives. You can use the power of plants to fuel your workouts, improve performance, and nourish your body if you have access to the correct equipment and ingredients.

The secret to vegan culinary success is having a well-stocked pantry, which offers a wealth of products that can be used to create a variety of tasty and nourishing dishes. Have a pantry full of basic ingredients so that you always have the ingredients on hand to make fulfilling recipes that please the palate and the body, regardless of how experienced you are with plant-based cooking.

Legumes, grains, and beans are the foundation of any vegan pantry; they are nutrient-dense powerhouses that can be used in a plethora of dishes. Packed in protein, these adaptable alternatives can be used in anything from substantial stews and salads to protein-packed burgers and breakfast bowls. Stock up on chickpeas, black beans, lentils, quinoa, rice, and oats. In addition to being reasonably priced and shelf-stable, these pantry essentials are also a great source of fiber, protein, and vital vitamins and minerals that will support your active lifestyle and nourish your body.

To add diversity and taste to your meals, a well-rounded vegan pantry should have a selection of plant-based proteins and meat substitutes in addition to grains and legumes. Look for plant-based burger patties such as tofu, tempeh, seitan, and others that can be marinated, seasoned, and cooked in a variety of ways to resemble the flavor and texture of meat. These high-protein choices provide a tasty substitute for conventional animal products and go well with stir-fries, sandwiches, tacos, and other dishes.

Without a variety of herbs, spices, and condiments to enhance your food and add complexity to your taste, no vegan pantry would be complete. Pantry essentials like soy sauce, tahini, vinegar, and plant-based milk provide richness and umami to a range of dishes, while essentials like garlic, onions, ginger, cumin, paprika, and nutritional yeast are invaluable for flavoring soups, sauces, marinades, and salads.

Remember to have a variety of nuts, seeds, and dried fruits on hand for baking, nibbling, and incorporating into your meals to give them crunch and texture. Nutrient-dense nuts and seeds, such as walnuts, chia seeds, and pumpkin seeds, combine well with yogurt, porridge, and salads. They may also be used for homemade granola, energy bars, and trail mixes for convenient on-the-go energy.

Keeping these vegan essentials in your cupboard will ensure that you're always ready to make scrumptious and nourishing meals that fulfill your desires, energize your exercise, and nurture your body from the inside out. You can make delicious and fulfilling vegan meals that delight your palate and promote your health and well-being with a little imagination and a well-stocked pantry.

Having the correct tools and equipment is essential for vegan bodybuilders who want to master the kitchen. It's like having the ideal workout music when it comes to success; it sets the tone for your culinary journey and makes all the difference.

Imagine yourself entering your kitchen with a goal in mind and your best apron on. But let's speak about the necessary tools that will make your culinary fantasies come true before you get started preparing your culinary masterpieces.

Let's start by discussing the all-powerful blender. Your pass to silky sauces, velvety soups, and creamy smoothies is this culinary powerhouse. A high-speed blender is essential whether you're making a batch of delicious cashew cheese or churning up a post-workout protein drink. You will question how you ever survived without a high-quality blender once you've experienced its brilliance, I promise.

A good pair of knives is the next item on the list. Investing in high-quality knives is vital for vegan bodybuilders since they will be slicing and chopping a plethora of fresh fruits and vegetables. A good blade is your greatest buddy in the kitchen, whether you're cutting precisely or delicately julienning. Plus, there's something very fulfilling about the rhythmic action of cutting vegetables—it works your hands like a little exercise!

Let's now discuss kitchenware. A multifunctional cast-iron skillet is a must-have in my kitchen. It not only gives a delicate depth of flavor to your food, but it also distributes heat evenly for flawless sears and sautés. A reliable cast-iron pan will never fail you down, whether you're cooking a delicious portobello steak or making a substantial tofu scramble.

Let's now discuss kitchenware. A multifunctional cast-iron skillet is a must-have in my kitchen. It not only gives a delicate depth of flavor to your food, but it also distributes heat evenly for flawless sears and sautés. A reliable cast-iron pan will never fail you down, whether you're cooking a delicious portobello steak or making a substantial tofu scramble.

Of course, without a trustworthy food processor, no kitchen arsenal is complete. A food processor brings you a world of culinary possibilities, from pounding oats into flour for protein-packed pancakes to blitzing nuts and seeds into velvety nut butter. It's like having a personal sous chef at your disposal who can quickly and precisely handle any assignment.

Let's speak about storage containers last but most definitely not least. Meal planning is essential if you're a vegan bodybuilder who wants to maintain your dietary targets. Purchasing a set of sturdy, airtight containers can guarantee that your food is tasty and fresh for the whole week. Having the appropriate containers on hand can expedite your meal prep process and position you for success, whether you're keeping prepared vegetables, batch-cooked grains, or ready-to-eat meals.

That's my list of essential kitchen utensils and equipment for successful vegan bodybuilding. Armed with these fundamentals, you'll be prepared to approach any dish with courage and inventiveness. Let's cook tasty, wholesome meals that nourish your body and your spirit.

Meal preparation is more than just a job for a vegan bodybuilder; it's a game-changer that paves the way for success both inside and outside the gym. Allow me to share with you some exclusive secrets and methods that have completely changed the way I nourish my body with delicious plant-based foods.

Plan Like a Pro: Take some time to schedule your meals for the next week before you go in the kitchen. Take into account your nutritional objectives, training plan, and any impending activities that may have an impact on your eating habits. You may stay away from last-minute scrambles and make sure you have all the supplies you need on hand by making a clear strategy in advance.

Keep It Simple: When it comes to efficient meal preparation, keeping things simple is essential, despite the allure of complex gourmet dinners. Pay attention to dishes that are simple to make in large quantities and that retain taste and texture whether refrigerated or frozen. Imagine substantial dishes like stir-fries, grain bowls, and soups that are high in nutrients yet don't take a lot of time to prepare.

Accept Batch Cooking: Batch cooking is one of the ways I save the most time while preparing meals. I can make many variants of filling meals throughout the week by making huge amounts of essentials like grains, beans, and roasted veggies ahead of time. Keeping ingredients on hand also simplifies the process of preparing wholesome meals quickly on hectic days.

Invest in High-Quality Containers: Storing your made foods correctly will keep them tasting and remaining fresh. Purchase a set of premium, microwave-safe, long-lasting, and leak-proof containers. To reduce your influence on the environment and guarantee that your food remains safe and nutritious, use glass or BPA-free plastic alternatives.

Be Creative with taste: Don't be scared to experiment with taste; eating the same thing every day might grow boring very soon. Try varying the herbs, spices, and condiments you use to add flavor and excitement to your food. There are many ways to enhance your vegan dishes, ranging from spicy dressings to creamy sauces and sour marinades.

Keep Your Kitchen Organized: Any effective meal prep enthusiast's hidden weapon is a well-kept kitchen. To prevent misunderstanding and waste, take the effort to mark your containers with the contents and date. Assign dedicated spaces for food preparation, cooking, and storage, and keep your pantry full of necessities like grains, beans, and spices.

Create a Ritual: Lastly, recognize that preparing meals is a ritual that involves both self-care and feeding. Allocate a certain period each week to concentrate on cooking and consuming healthful meals that feed your body and spirit. Enjoy a cup of tea, turn on your favorite podcast or music, and let the calming sound of chopping, stirring, and boiling to bring you back to the present.

You'll save time and money by implementing these meal prep strategies into your routine, and you'll also position yourself for success in your vegan bodybuilding endeavors. Now let's start cooking, put on your sleeves, polish your knives.

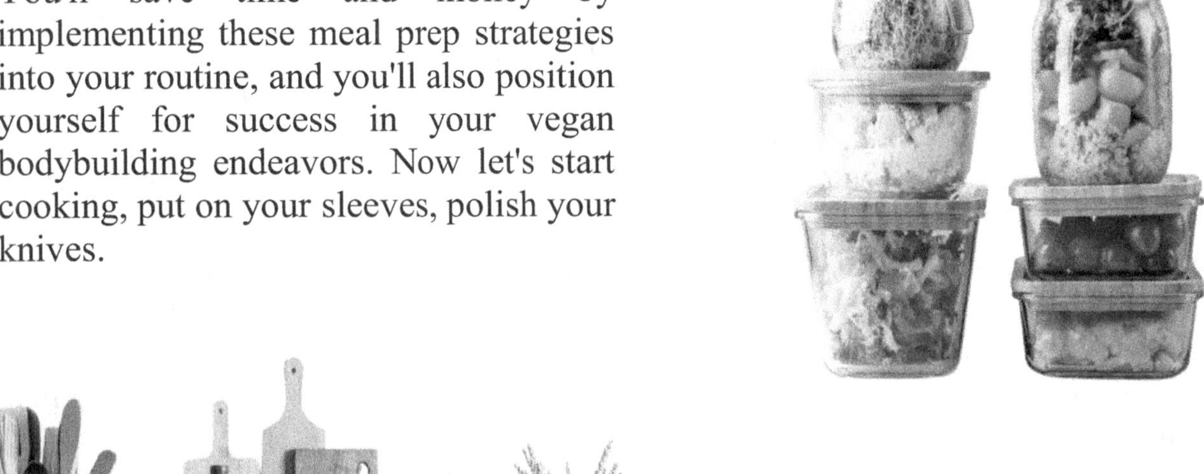

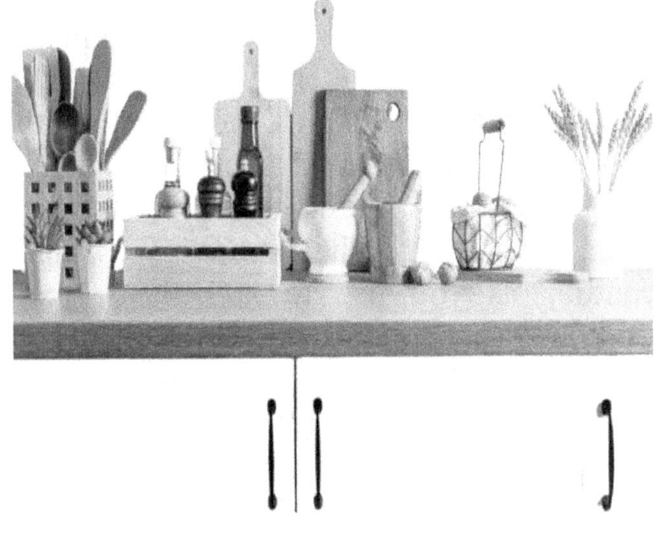

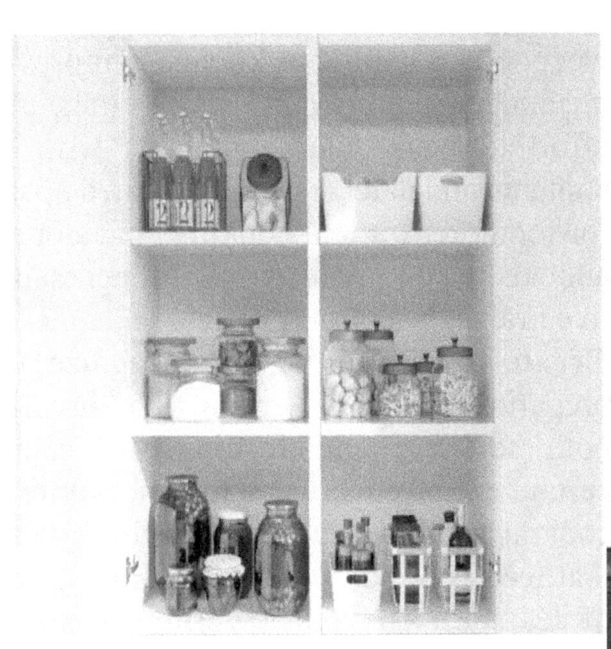

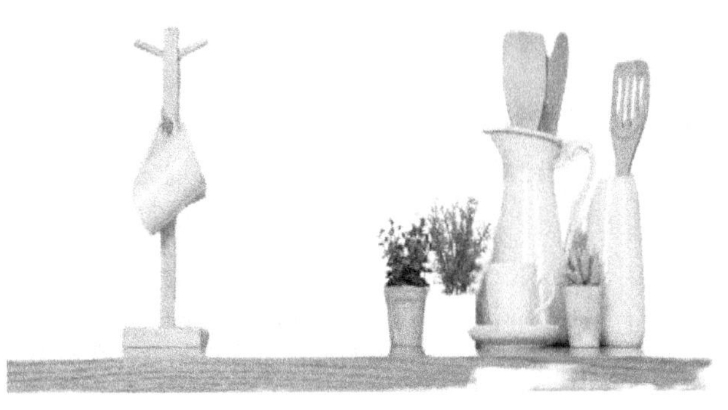

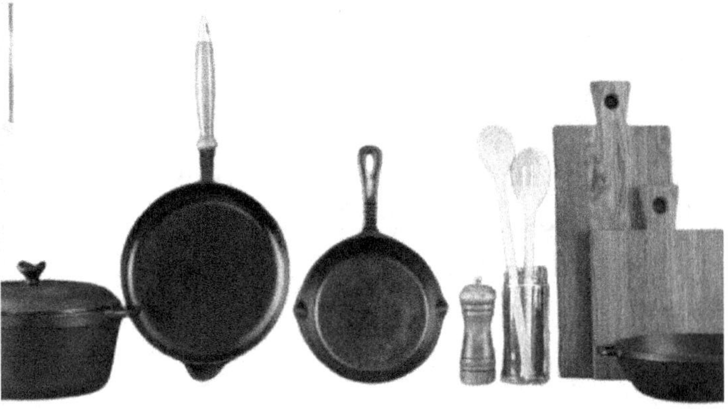

Chapter 1

BREAKFAST POWERHOUSES

High-Protein Smoothie Bowl with Berries Blast

INGREDIENTS

- ❖ One cup of frozen berry mixture (raspberries, blueberries, and strawberries)
- ❖ One ripe banana
- ❖ One scoop of berry- or vanilla-flavored vegan protein powder
- ❖ Half a cup of unflavored almond milk
- ❖ One spoonful of chia seeds
- ❖ Toppers: chopped coconut, granola, fresh berries, and banana slices

PREPARATION

- ❖ Blend together the frozen mixed berries, ripe banana, almond milk, vegan protein powder, and chia seeds using a blender.
- ❖ To get the right consistency, add more almond milk if necessary and blend until smooth and creamy.
- ❖ After transferring the smoothie into a bowl, garnish it with shredded coconut, granola, fresh berries, and banana slices.
- ❖ Savor it right away for a filling and tasty breakfast or lunch after working out!

Nutrition Information

- ➤ Serving size: one dish
- ➤ 350 calories
- ➤ 25g of protein
- ➤ 45g of carbohydrates
- ➤ 7g of fat
- ➤ 12g of fiber
- ➤ Five minutes for preparation
- ➤ Time Spent Cooking: 0 minutes

Protein-Rich Tropical Paradise Smoothie Bowl

INGREDIENTS

- ❖ One cup of frozen pineapple chunks
- ❖ Half a cup of frozen mango chunks
- ❖ One ripe banana
- ❖ 1 scoop vanilla or tropical-flavored vegan protein powder
- ❖ half a cup of coconut water
- ❖ One spoonful of hemp seeds
- ❖ Sliced kiwi, shredded coconut, chopped almonds, and chia seeds are the toppings.

PREPARATION

- ❖ Blend together the frozen pineapple and mango pieces, ripe banana, hemp seeds, vegan protein powder, and coconut water in a blender.
- ❖ To get the right consistency, add more coconut water if necessary and blend until smooth and creamy.
- ❖ Transfer the smoothie into a bowl and garnish with chia seeds, chopped almonds, shredded coconut, and sliced kiwi.
- ❖ Savor the revitalizing tastes of this tropical pleasure while you provide your body with nutrients and plant-powered protein!

Nutrition Information

- ➤ Serving size: one dish
- ➤ 380 calories
- ➤ 20g of protein
- ➤ 55g of carbohydrates
- ➤ 10g of fat
- ➤ 10g of fiber
- ➤ Five minutes for preparation
- ➤ Time Spent Cooking: 0 minutes

The High-Protein Smoothie Bowl by Green Goddess

INGREDIENTS

- ❖ two cups of raw spinach
- ❖ One mature avocado
- ❖ One ripe banana
- ❖ One scoop of vanilla or unflavored vegan protein powder
- ❖ Half a cup of unflavored almond milk
- ❖ One spoonful of butter made with almonds
- ❖ Slicing kiwi, hemp seeds, sliced almonds, and pumpkin seeds are the toppings.

PREPARATION

- ❖ Blend together the fresh spinach, ripe avocado, ripe banana, almond milk, vegan protein powder, and almond butter using a blender.
- ❖ Add extra almond milk as necessary to alter the consistency after blending until it's smooth and creamy.
- ❖ Transfer the smoothie into a bowl and garnish with sliced almonds, pumpkin seeds, hemp seeds, and kiwi slices.
- ❖ Savor this nutrient-dense green goddess dish, which is full of vitamins, healthy fats, and protein to help your body function at its best!

Nutrition Information

- ➢ Serving size: one dish
- ➢ 420 calories
- ➢ 22g of protein
- ➢ 35g of carbohydrates
- ➢ 25g of fat
- ➢ 15g of fiber
- ➢ Five minutes for preparation
- ➢ Time Spent Cooking: 0 minutes

Filling Burritos for Breakfast

INGREDIENTS

- ❖ One cup of cooked quinoa
- ❖ One cup of rinsed and drained black beans
- ❖ one cup of tempeh or tofu, diced
- ❖ One chopped bell pepper
- ❖ One chopped onion
- ❖ One teaspoon of cumin powder
- ❖ One tsp of chili powder
- ❖ To taste, add salt and pepper.
- ❖ Four big tortillas made with whole wheat
- ❖ One sliced avocado
- ❖ For garnish, use fresh cilantro.
- ❖ Hot sauce or salsa are optional

PREPARATION

- ❖ Add the chopped onion and bell pepper to a pan and cook over medium heat until they become tender.
- ❖ Cook the diced tempeh or tofu in the pan until it begins to color slightly.
- ❖ Add the black beans, ground cumin, chili powder, cooked quinoa, salt, and pepper. Cook for a further two to three minutes, or until well heated.
- ❖ To make the whole wheat tortillas more malleable, briefly warm them in the pan or microwave.
- ❖ Spoon the filling in the middle of each tortilla after dividing it equally among them.
- ❖ Add sliced avocado and fresh cilantro to the top of each tortilla.
- ❖ Enclose the filling by firmly rolling the tortillas and tucking in the sides as you roll.
- ❖ If preferred, serve right now with salsa or spicy sauce on the side.

Nutrition Information

- ➢ Size of Serving: One Burrito
- ➢ 350 calories
- ➢ 15g of protein
- ➢ 45g of carbohydrates
- ➢ 10g of fiber
- ➢ 12g of fat
- ➢ Ten minutes for preparation
- ➢ 15 minutes is the cooking time.

Breakfast burritos with spinach and mushrooms

INGREDIENTS

- ❖ One cup of brown rice, cooked
- ❖ one cup of finely chopped spinach
- ❖ One cup of sliced mushrooms
- ❖ One teaspoon garlic powder, half a cup sliced onion, and half a cup diced bell pepper
- ❖ Half a teaspoon of paprika
- ❖ To taste, add salt and pepper.
- ❖ Four big tortillas made with whole wheat
- ❖ Half a cup of vegan cheese, shredded (optional)
- ❖ Hot sauce or salsa are optional.

PREPARATION

- ❖ Add the chopped onion and bell pepper to a pan and cook over medium heat until they become tender.
- ❖ Sliced mushrooms should be added to the pan and cooked until they release moisture and soften.
- ❖ Add the cooked brown rice, chopped spinach, paprika, garlic powder, salt, and pepper. Cook the spinach for a further two to three minutes, or until it wilts.
- ❖ To make the whole wheat tortillas more malleable, briefly warm them in the pan or microwave.
- ❖ Spoon the filling in the middle of each tortilla after dividing it equally among them.
- ❖ Top the filling with shredded vegan cheese, if using.
- ❖ Enclose the filling by firmly rolling the tortillas and tucking in the sides as you roll.
- ❖ If preferred, serve right now with salsa or spicy sauce on the side.

Nutrition Information

- ➢ Size of Serving: One Burrito
- ➢ 300 calories
- ➢ 10g of protein
- ➢ 45g of carbohydrates
- ➢ 8g of fiber
- ➢ 8g of fat
- ➢ Ten minutes for preparation
- ➢ 15 minutes is the cooking time.

Breakfast Burritos with Sweet Potato and Black Beans

INGREDIENTS

- ❖ Two cups of cooked, mashed sweet potatoes
- ❖ One cup of cooked, rinsed and drained black beans
- ❖ half a cup of red onion, chopped
- ❖ half a cup of finely chopped cilantro
- ❖ One teaspoon of cumin powder
- ❖ One tsp of smoky paprika
- ❖ To taste, add salt and pepper.
- ❖ Four big tortillas made with whole wheat
- ❖ Half a cup of sliced avocado
- ❖ slices of lime, for serving

PREPARATION

- ❖ Mashed sweet potato, cooked black beans, sliced red onion, chopped cilantro, smoked paprika, ground cumin, and salt and pepper should all be properly blended in a big bowl.
- ❖ To make the whole wheat tortillas more malleable, briefly warm them in the pan or microwave.
- ❖ Spread the black bean and sweet potato mixture evenly in the middle of each tortilla after dividing it equally among them.
- ❖ Place a sliced avocado on top of each tortilla.
- ❖ Enclose the filling by firmly rolling the tortillas and tucking in the sides as you roll.
- ❖ Serve right away, squeezing lime wedges over the burritos from the side.

Nutrition Information

- ➢ Size of Serving: One Burrito
- ➢ 320 calories
- ➢ 10g of protein
- ➢ 50g of carbohydrates
- ➢ 10g of fiber
- ➢ 8g of fat
- ➢ 15 minutes for preparation
- ➢ 15 minutes is the cooking time.

Breakfast Burritos with Tofu Scramble

INGREDIENTS

- ❖ One block of extra-firm, crushed and drained tofu
- ❖ one cup of bell peppers, chopped
- ❖ One cup each of chopped onion and spinach
- ❖ two minced garlic cloves
- ❖ One tsp of turmeric
- ❖ half a teaspoon of cumin powder
- ❖ To taste, add salt and pepper.
- ❖ Four big tortillas made with whole wheat
- ❖ half a cup of salsa
- ❖ 1/4 cup (optional) nutritional yeast

PREPARATION

- ❖ Add the chopped onion and bell pepper to a pan and cook over medium heat until they become tender.
- ❖ When the garlic is fragrant, return it to the pan with the minced garlic and cook for one more minute.
- ❖ Toss in the crushed tofu, turmeric, ground cumin, salt, and pepper in the skillet. Cook, stirring periodically, until the tofu is well cooked and beginning to turn brown, 5 to 7 minutes.
- ❖ Cook the chopped spinach for a further two to three minutes, or until it wilts.
- ❖ To make the whole wheat tortillas more malleable, briefly warm them in the pan or microwave.
- ❖ Spoon the tofu scramble in the middle of each tortilla, dividing it equally among them.
- ❖ Place some salsa and, if using, nutritional yeast on top of each tortilla.
- ❖ Enclose the filling by firmly rolling the tortillas and tucking in the sides as you roll.
- ❖ Serve right now, or cover with foil for an easy breakfast to go.

Nutrition Information

- ➢ Size of Serving: One Burrito
- ➢ 280 calories
- ➢ 15g of protein
- ➢ 30g of carbohydrates
- ➢ 8g of fiber
- ➢ 10g of fat
- ➢ Ten minutes for preparation
- ➢ 15 minutes is the cooking time.

Burritos with spinach and chickpeas for breakfast

INGREDIENTS

- ❖ One can of washed and drained chickpeas
- ❖ 1/2 cup sliced onion, 1/2 cup diced bell pepper, and 1 cup chopped spinach
- ❖ two minced garlic cloves
- ❖ One teaspoon of cumin powder
- ❖ One-half tsp smoked paprika
- ❖ To taste, add salt and pepper.
- ❖ Four big tortillas made with whole wheat
- ❖ 1/4 cup finely chopped fresh parsley and 1/2 cup hummus

PREPARATION

- ❖ Add the chopped onion and bell pepper to a pan and cook over medium heat until they become tender.
- ❖ When the garlic is fragrant, return it to the pan with the minced garlic and cook for one more minute.
- ❖ Add the smoked paprika, ground cumin, salt, and pepper to the pan with the chickpeas. Cook, tossing periodically, until the chickpeas are cooked through and beginning to crisp up, 5 to 7 minutes.
- ❖ Cook the chopped spinach for a further two to three minutes, or until it wilts.
- ❖ To make the whole wheat tortillas more malleable, briefly warm them in the pan or microwave.
- ❖ On each tortilla, generously spread a layer of hummus.
- ❖ Spoon the combination of chickpeas and spinach in the middle of each tortilla, dividing it equally between them.
- ❖ Top the contents with a few chopped fresh parsley strands.
- ❖ Enclose the filling by firmly rolling the tortillas and tucking in the sides as you roll.
- ❖ Serve right now, or cover with foil for an easy breakfast to go.

Nutrition Information

- ➢ Size of Serving: One Burrito
- ➢ 310 calories
- ➢ 12g of protein
- ➢ 45g of carbohydrates
- ➢ 10g of fiber
- ➢ 8g of fat
- ➢ Ten minutes for preparation
- ➢ 15 minutes is the cooking time.

Sausage and Vegan Breakfast Burritos

INGREDIENTS

- ❖ Four sausages for breakfast that are vegan
- ❖ one cup of bell peppers, chopped
- ❖ One cup cooked quinoa and one cup chopped onion
- ❖ half a cup of freshly chopped parsley
- ❖ To taste, add salt and pepper.
- ❖ Four big tortillas made with whole wheat
- ❖ 1/2 cup of cheese shreds without dairy
- ❖ Hot sauce or salsa are optional.

PREPARATION

- ❖ Follow the directions on the box to prepare the vegan breakfast sausages. Cut them into bite-sized pieces once they're cooked.
- ❖ Add the chopped onion and bell pepper to a pan and cook over medium heat until they become tender.
- ❖ Add the cooked quinoa, salt, pepper, and freshly chopped parsley. Cook for a further two to three minutes, or until well heated.
- ❖ To make the whole wheat tortillas more malleable, briefly warm them in the pan or microwave.
- ❖ Spoon the quinoa mixture into the middle of each tortilla, dividing it equally between them.
- ❖ Place sliced vegan breakfast sausages and dairy-free cheese shreds on top of each tortilla.
- ❖ Enclose the filling by firmly rolling the tortillas and tucking in the sides as you roll.
- ❖ If preferred, serve right now with salsa or spicy sauce on the side.

Nutrition Information

- ➤ Size of Serving: One Burrito
- ➤ 380 calories
- ➤ 15g of protein
- ➤ 45g of carbohydrates
- ➤ 8g of fiber
- ➤ 15g of fat
- ➤ Ten minutes for preparation
- ➤ 15 minutes is the cooking time.

Breakfast burritos with peanut butter and banana

INGREDIENTS

- ❖ Four big tortillas made with whole wheat
- ❖ Half a cup of natural peanut butter
- ❖ Two bananas, cut thinly
- ❖ 1/4 cup of finely chopped nuts, such walnuts or almonds
- ❖ 1/4 cup dried cranberries or raisins
- ❖ Two teaspoons (optional) of maple syrup
- ❖ Cinnamon, ground, to be sprinkled

PREPARATION

- ❖ Generous amounts of peanut butter should be spread over each whole wheat tortilla.
- ❖ Place the bananas, thinly sliced, over the peanut butter.
- ❖ Over the bananas, scatter chopped almonds, raisins, or dried cranberries.
- ❖ If using, drizzle maple syrup over the filling.
- ❖ To taste, sprinkle ground cinnamon on top of the filling.
- ❖ Enclose the filling by firmly rolling the tortillas and tucking in the sides as you roll.
- ❖ Serve right now, or cover with foil for an easy breakfast to go.

Nutrition Information

- ➤ Size of Serving: One Burrito
- ➤ 400 calories
- ➤ 10g of protein
- ➤ 50g of carbohydrates
- ➤ 8g of fiber
- ➤ 18g of fat
- ➤ Five minutes for preparation
- ➤ Time Spent Cooking: 0 minutes

Chapter 2

HEARTY LUNCHES FOR MUSCLE FUEL

Quinoa and Chickpea Power Bowl

INGREDIENTS

- ❖ One cup of cooked quinoa
- ❖ One can of washed and drained chickpeas
- ❖ One cup of chopped mixed veggies, including tomatoes, cucumbers, and bell peppers
- ❖ Two teaspoons of freshly chopped parsley
- ❖ One lemon's juice
- ❖ To taste, add salt and pepper.

PREPARATION

- ❖ The cooked quinoa, chickpeas, mixed veggies, and parsley should all be combined in a big dish.
- ❖ Sprinkle salt and pepper on top of the mixture and drizzle with lemon juice.
- ❖ Mix everything until well incorporated.
- ❖ Serve right now or store in the fridge for later.

Nutrition Information

- ➢ 15g of protein
- ➢ 40g of carbohydrates
- ➢ 5g of fat
- ➢ 10g of fiber
- ➢ Ten minutes for preparation
- ➢ No cooking time

Stir-fried Tofu with Veggies

INGREDIENTS

- ❖ One block of pressed and diced extra-firm tofu
- ❖ Two cups of mixed veggies, such as bell peppers, broccoli, and snap peas
- ❖ Two tsp soy sauce
- ❖ One tablespoon of sesame oil
- ❖ one tsp finely chopped garlic
- ❖ Prepared quinoa or brown rice for serving

PREPARATION

- ❖ In a large skillet over medium heat, warm the sesame oil. When aromatic, add the minced garlic and simmer.
- ❖ When the cubed tofu is golden brown on both sides, add it to the skillet.
- ❖ To the skillet, add the mixed veggies and soy sauce. Stir-fry the veggies until they become crisp-tender.
- ❖ Serve the cooked quinoa or brown rice with the tofu and veggie stir-fry.

Nutrition Information

- ➢ 20g of protein
- ➢ 30g of carbohydrates
- ➢ 10g of fat
- ➢ 8g of fiber
- ➢ 15 minutes for preparation
- ➢ 15 minutes is the cooking time.

Burrito Bowl with Sweet Potato and Black Beans

INGREDIENTS

- ❖ One cup of black beans, cooked
- ❖ One big sweet potato, cut into pieces and baked
- ❖ One cup of brown rice, cooked
- ❖ One cup of finely chopped lettuce
- ❖ Avocado, salsa, and vegan sour cream as garnish

PREPARATION

- ❖ Spoon cooked black beans, cooked brown rice, roasted sweet potato, and shredded lettuce into serving dishes.
- ❖ Add vegan sour cream, guacamole, and salsa to the top of each bowl.
- ❖ Combine all ingredients and serve.

Nutrition Information

- ➢ 18g of protein
- ➢ 50g of carbohydrates
- ➢ 8g of fat
- ➢ 12g of fiber
- ➢ Twenty minutes for preparation
- ➢ Cooking time for sweet potatoes is thirty minutes.

Tempeh BLT Wrap

INGREDIENTS

- ❖ One container of sliced tempeh and four whole wheat wraps
- ❖ One cup of sliced cherry tomatoes and two cups of shredded lettuce
- ❖ One avocado, cut into slices, with vegan mayonnaise or hummus to spread

PREPARATION

- ❖ A nonstick skillet should be heated to medium heat. Cook the tempeh slices until they get golden brown on both sides.
- ❖ Arrange the whole wheat wrappers and top with a dollop of vegan hummus or mayonnaise.
- ❖ Top each wrap with a portion of cooked tempeh, avocado, shredded lettuce, and cherry tomatoes.
- ❖ Before serving, securely roll the wraps and cut in half.

Nutrition Information

- ➢ 22g of protein
- ➢ 40g of carbohydrates
- ➢ 15g of fat
- ➢ 10g of fiber
- ➢ 15 minutes for preparation
- ➢ Ten minutes to cook

Black bean and Quinoa Stuffed Peppers

INGREDIENTS

- ❖ Four big bell peppers, seeded and halved
- ❖ One cup cooked black beans and one cup cooked quinoa
- ❖ One cup of kernel corn
- ❖ one cup of tomatoes, chopped
- ❖ One tsp of chili powder
- ❖ One teaspoon of cumin
- ❖ To taste, add salt and pepper.

PREPARATION

- ❖ Turn the oven on to 375°F, or 190°C.
- ❖ Cooked quinoa, black beans, corn kernels, chopped tomatoes, cumin, chili powder, salt, and pepper should all be combined in a big dish.
- ❖ Place the black bean and quinoa mixture into each half of a bell pepper.
- ❖ Cover the filled peppers with foil after placing them in a roasting dish. Bake peppers for 25 to 30 minutes, or until soft.
- ❖ If desired, top hot dish with diced avocado or cilantro.

Nutrition Information

- ➢ 16g of protein
- ➢ 35g of carbohydrates
- ➢ 3g of fat
- ➢ Fiber: nine grams
- ➢ Twenty minutes for preparation
- ➢ 30 minutes for cooking

Lentil Chili for Vegans

INGREDIENTS

- ❖ one cup of washed and dried green lentils
- ❖ One can of chopped tomatoes
- ❖ One can of washed and drained kidney beans
- ❖ One chopped onion, two minced garlic cloves, and one diced bell pepper
- ❖ One tablespoon of powdered chilies
- ❖ One teaspoon of cumin
- ❖ To taste, add salt and pepper.

PREPARATION

- ❖ Heat a little amount of olive oil in a big saucepan over medium heat. Add the chopped bell pepper, minced garlic, and onion. Simmer until tender.
- ❖ To the saucepan, add the kidney beans, chopped tomatoes, cumin, chili powder, salt, and pepper.
- ❖ Bring the mixture to a boil by adding enough water to cover the contents.
- ❖ Once the lentils are soft and the chili has thickened, reduce heat and simmer for around half an hour.
- ❖ If desired, top hot dish with chopped green onions or cilantro.

Nutrition Information

- ➢ 20g of protein
- ➢ 45g of carbohydrates
- ➢ Fat: 1 gram
- ➢ 15g of fiber
- ➢ 15 minutes for preparation
- ➢ 40 minutes for cooking
- ➢

Hummus and Veggie Wrap

INGREDIENTS

- ❖ Four wraps made entirely with whole wheat
- ❖ One cup of hummus
- ❖ two cups of mixed greens for salad
- ❖ One cucumber, cut thinly
- ❖ One bell pepper, cut thinly
- ❖ half a cup of carrots, shredded
- ❖ Microgreens or sprouts as a garnish

PREPARATION

- ❖ Put some hummus on each whole wheat wrapper.
- ❖ Spoon sliced bell pepper, sliced cucumber, shredded carrots, and mixed salad greens among the wraps.
- ❖ Add microgreens or sprouts to the top of each wrap.
- ❖ Before serving, securely roll the wraps and cut in half.

Nutrition Information

- ➤ 12g of protein
- ➤ 40g of carbohydrates
- ➤ 8g of fat
- ➤ 10g of fiber
- ➤ Ten minutes for preparation
- ➤ No cooking time

Buddha Bowl with Sweet Potato and Lentil

INGREDIENTS

- ❖ One cup of cooked quinoa or brown rice
- ❖ One big sweet potato, cut into pieces and baked
- ❖ One cup of cooked green lentils
- ❖ two cups of mixed greens
- ❖ Slicing 1/4 cup of almonds
- ❖ Tahini dressing or balsamic vinaigrette to drizzle

PREPARATION

- ❖ Spoon cooked brown rice or quinoa, cooked green lentils, roasted sweet potato, and mixed greens into individual serving dishes.
- ❖ Place sliced almonds over the top of every bowl.
- ❖ Before serving, drizzle with tahini dressing or balsamic vinaigrette

Nutrition Information

- ➤ 18g of protein
- ➤ 45g of carbohydrates
- ➤ 10g of fat
- ➤ 12g of fiber
- ➤ Twenty minutes for preparation
- ➤ Cooking time for sweet potatoes is thirty minutes.

Barbecue without meat Sandwich with Jackfruit

INGREDIENTS

- ❖ One can of young, green, brine-drained, and shredded jackfruit
- ❖ half a cup barbecue sauce
- ❖ Burger buns: 4 whole grain buns
- ❖ Coleslaw as a garnish, if desired

PREPARATION

- ❖ In a pan, thoroughly cook the shredded jackfruit and BBQ sauce over medium heat.
- ❖ If preferred, toast whole grain burger buns.
- ❖ Spoon the Barbecued Jackfruit mixture onto each burger bun.
- ❖ If desired, top with coleslaw before serving.

Nutrition Information

- ➢ 10g of protein
- ➢ 50g of carbohydrates
- ➢ 3g of fat
- ➢ 8g of fiber
- ➢ Ten minutes for preparation
- ➢ Ten minutes to cook

Mediterranean Salad with Chickpeas

INGREDIENTS

- ❖ two cups of boiled lentils
- ❖ one cup of cucumbers, chopped
- ❖ Half a cup of cherry tomatoes
- ❖ 1/4 cup of red onion, chopped
- ❖ 1/4 cup of freshly chopped parsley
- ❖ One lemon's juice
- ❖ Two teaspoons pure olive oil
- ❖ One tsp of dehydrated oregano
- ❖ To taste, add salt and pepper.

PREPARATION

- ❖ The cooked chickpeas, sliced cucumber, cherry tomatoes, diced red onion, and chopped fresh parsley should all be combined in a big bowl.
- ❖ Over the mixture, drizzle extra virgin olive oil and lemon juice.
- ❖ Season the salad with salt, pepper, and dry oregano.
- ❖ Mix everything until well incorporated.
- ❖ Serve right now or store in the fridge for later.

Nutrition Information

- ➢ 15g of protein
- ➢ 30g of carbohydrates
- ➢ 10g of fat
- ➢ 10g of fiber
- ➢ 15 minutes for preparation
- ➢ No cooking time

Chapter 3

POST-WORKOUT RECOVERY MEALS

Black bean and Quinoa Salad

INGREDIENTS

- One cup of quinoa
- One can of washed and drained black beans
- One chopped bell pepper
- Half a cup of cherry tomatoes
- 1/4 cup of coarsely chopped red onion
- Two teaspoons of freshly cut cilantro
- one lime's juice
- To taste, add salt and pepper.

PREPARATION

- As directed on the box, prepare the quinoa and let it to cool.
- Cooked quinoa, black beans, bell pepper, cherry tomatoes, red onion, and cilantro should all be combined in a big dish.
- Pour lime juice over the salad and mix everything together. To taste, add salt and pepper for seasoning.

Nutrition Information

- 350 calories
- 15g of protein
- 60g of carbohydrates
- 5g of fat
- Ten minutes for preparation
- 20 minutes for cooking

Stir-fried Tofu with Vegetables

INGREDIENTS

- 1 block diced and pressed extra-firm tofu
- Two cups of mixed veggies, including carrots, snap peas, broccoli, and bell peppers
- three minced garlic cloves
- Two tsp soy sauce
- One tablespoon of sesame oil
- One spoonful of maple syrup
- cooked quinoa or brown rice, ready to be served

PREPARATION

- In a large skillet over medium heat, warm the sesame oil. Tofu cubes should be added and cooked until golden brown all over. Take out the tofu and put it aside in a skillet.
- Add mixed veggies and minced garlic to the same skillet. Stir-fry the veggies until they become crisp-tender.
- Put the tofu back in the pan along with the maple syrup and soy sauce. Stirring to ensure that everything is uniformly coated, cook for a further two to three minutes.
- Serve stir-fried rice or quinoa that has been cooked.

Nutrition Information

- 400 calories
- 25g of protein
- 45g of carbohydrates
- 15g of fat
- 15 minutes for preparation
- 15 minutes is the cooking time.

Curry with Chickpeas and Spinach

INGREDIENTS

- One tablespoon of coconut oil
- One chopped onion and three minced garlic cloves
- One tablespoon of finely chopped ginger
- One can of washed and drained chickpeas
- One can of chopped tomatoes
- two cups of spinach
- One can of coconut milk
- Curry powder, two teaspoons
- To taste, add salt and pepper

PREPARATION

- In a large saucepan set over medium heat, warm the coconut oil. Add the ginger, garlic, and sliced onion. Cook until onions become transparent and aromatic.
- Add the spinach, chopped tomatoes, chickpeas, coconut milk, and curry powder and stir. To taste, add salt and pepper for seasoning.
- Curry should be simmered for 15 to 20 minutes, stirring now and again, until the flavors are completely blended and the spinach has wilted.
- Curry should be served with cooked quinoa or brown rice.

Nutrition Information

- 380 calories
- 15g of protein
- 40g of carbohydrates
- 20g of fat
- Ten minutes for preparation
- 25 minutes for cooking

Soup with Protein-Packed Lentils

INGREDIENTS

- One tablespoon of olive oil
- One chopped onion and two diced carrots
- two chopped celery stalks
- three minced garlic cloves
- One cup of dehydrated green lentils
- Four cups of broth made with vegetables
- One can of chopped tomatoes
- two cups of spinach
- A single tsp of dried thyme
- To taste, add salt and pepper.

PREPARATION

- In a big saucepan, warm up the olive oil over medium heat. Add the celery, carrots, and chopped onion. Sauté the veggies till they get tender.
- Add the dried thyme and minced garlic. Simmer one more minute, or until aromatic.
- To the saucepan, add chopped tomatoes, vegetable broth, and dry lentils. Once the lentils are cooked, simmer for 20 to 25 minutes on low heat after bringing to a boil.
- Add the spinach and stir-fry until it wilts. To taste, add salt and pepper for seasoning.

Nutrition Information

- 320 calories
- 20g of protein
- 45g of carbohydrates
- 5g of fat
- Ten minutes for preparation
- 30 minutes for cooking

Banana and Peanut Butter Protein Smoothie

INGREDIENTS

- ❖ Two ripe bananas
- ❖ Two tsp of peanut butter
- ❖ 1 cup almond milk without sugar
- ❖ One scoop of plant-based protein powder
- ❖ One-third cup flaxseeds
- ❖ One tablespoon of maple syrup, if desired

PREPARATION

- ❖ In a blender, combine all ingredients and process until smooth and creamy.
- ❖ Add additional almond milk to the smoothie if it's too thick until the right consistency is achieved.
- ❖ Pour into cups and start drinking right away.

Nutrition Information

- ➢ 380 calories
- ➢ 25g of protein
- ➢ 45g of carbohydrates
- ➢ 15g of fat
- ➢ Five minutes for preparation
- ➢ Time Spent Cooking: 0 minutes

Tofu Scramble Packed with Protein

INGREDIENTS

- ❖ 1 block crumbled extra-firm tofu
- ❖ One tablespoon of olive oil
- ❖ One chopped bell pepper
- ❖ Half a cup of cherry tomatoes
- ❖ two cups of spinach
- ❖ One tsp of turmeric
- ❖ To taste, add salt and pepper.

PREPARATION

- ❖ In a big skillet over medium heat, warm up the olive oil. Cook the crushed tofu for five to seven minutes, stirring now and again.
- ❖ Add the turmeric, cherry tomatoes, and sliced bell pepper. Sauté the veggies for a further three to four minutes, or until they are soft.
- ❖ Cook the spinach in the skillet until it wilts. To taste, add salt and pepper for seasoning.
- ❖ Avocado slices or whole grain bread go well with tofu scramble.

Nutrition Information

- ➢ 320 calories
- ➢ 20g of protein
- ➢ 15g of carbohydrates
- ➢ 20g of fat
- ➢ Ten minutes for preparation
- ➢ 15 minutes is the cooking time.

High-Protein Chia Seed Pudding

INGREDIENTS

- ❖ 1/4 cup of chia seeds.
- ❖ 1 cup almond milk without sugar
- ❖ One spoonful of maple syrup
- ❖ Half a teaspoon of extract from vanilla
- ❖ Topping: fresh berries

PREPARATION

- ❖ Chia seeds, almond milk, maple syrup, and vanilla extract should all be combined in a mixing dish. Mix well to blend.
- ❖ Place a lid on the bowl and place it in the refrigerator for a minimum of two hours or overnight, or until the mixture takes on the consistency of pudding.
- ❖ Present the pudding with chia seeds and fresh berries on top.

Nutrition Information

- ➢ 250 calories
- ➢ 10g of protein
- ➢ 25g of carbohydrates
- ➢ 10g of fat
- ➢ Five minutes for preparation
- ➢ Time Spent Cooking: 0 minutes

Hummus with vegetables Close

INGREDIENTS

- ❖ One whole grain tortilla is the ingredient.
- ❖ Two tsp of hummus
- ❖ Half a cup of mixed veggies, including spinach, bell peppers, cucumbers, and carrots
- ❖ 1/4 cup of sprouting alfalfa
- ❖ To taste, add salt and pepper.

PREPARATION

- ❖ Evenly coat the whole grain tortilla with hummus.
- ❖ Arrange the alfalfa sprouts and mixed veggies in a layer over the hummus.
- ❖ To taste, add salt and pepper for seasoning.
- ❖ Tightly roll the tortilla, then cut it in half. Savor right now or package for easy transport.

Nutrition Information

- ➢ 300 calories
- ➢ 10g of protein
- ➢ 40g of carbohydrates
- ➢ 10g of fat
- ➢ Five minutes for preparation
- ➢ Time Spent Cooking: 0 minutes

High-Protein Tofu Buddha Bowl

INGREDIENTS

- ❖ 1 cup of quinoa, cooked
- ❖ One block of extra-firm, cubed, baked tofu
- ❖ One cup of mixed greens (arugula, spinach, and kale).
- ❖ half a cup of cooked lentils
- ❖ Half a cup of sweet potatoes, roasted
- ❖ One-fourth cup of sliced avocado
- ❖ dressing with tahini One tablespoon each of tahini, lemon juice, and maple syrup

PREPARATION

- ❖ In a bowl, combine the cooked quinoa, roasted sweet potatoes, chickpeas, baked tofu, mixed greens, and sliced avocado.
- ❖ Pour over some tahini dressing.
- ❖ Enjoy after gently tossing to blend.

Nutrition Information

- ➢ 450 calories
- ➢ 25g of protein
- ➢ 45g of carbohydrates
- ➢ 20g of fat
- ➢ Ten minutes for preparation
- ➢ 30 minutes for cooking

Corn and Black Bean Salad Packed with Protein

INGREDIENTS

- ❖ 1 can rinsed and drained black beans
- ❖ One cup of kernel corn
- ❖ One chopped bell pepper
- ❖ 1/4 cup of coarsely chopped red onion
- ❖ 1/4 cup finely chopped fresh cilantro
- ❖ one lime's juice
- ❖ One tablespoon of olive oil
- ❖ To taste, add salt and pepper.

PREPARATION

- ❖ Black beans, corn kernels, chopped bell pepper, red onion, and cilantro should all be combined in a big dish.
- ❖ Pour lime juice and olive oil over the salad. To taste, add salt and pepper for seasoning.
- ❖ Before serving, toss to mix and let marinate for at least fifteen minutes.

Nutrition Information

- ➢ 300 calories
- ➢ 15g of protein
- ➢ 50g of carbohydrates
- ➢ 5g of fat
- ➢ Ten minutes for preparation
- ➢ Time Spent Cooking: 0 minutes

Chapter 4

MUSCLE-BUILDING DINNERS

Kale Chickpea Steak

INGREDIENTS

- ❖ two cups of boiled lentils
- ❖ One chopped onion
- ❖ two minced garlic cloves
- ❖ One chopped bell pepper
- ❖ one cup of tomatoes, chopped
- ❖ One cup coconut milk
- ❖ Curry powder, two teaspoons
- ❖ One tablespoon of coconut oil
- ❖ To taste, add salt and pepper.
- ❖ To garnish, use fresh cilantro.

PREPARATION

- ❖ In a large pan set over medium heat, warm the coconut oil. Sauté the chopped onion and garlic until they become transparent.
- ❖ Cook the chopped bell pepper until it becomes tender.
- ❖ After adding the curry powder, simmer for an additional minute.
- ❖ Add the cooked chickpeas and diced tomatoes. Mix well to blend.
- ❖ Add the coconut milk and cook the curry for ten to fifteen minutes, or until it thickens.
- ❖ To taste, add salt and pepper for seasoning.

Nutrition Information

- ➢ Serving size: one dish
- ➢ 320 calories
- ➢ 14g of protein
- ➢ 35g of carbohydrates
- ➢ 15g of fat
- ➢ 8g of fiber
- ➢ Ten minutes for preparation
- ➢ 20 minutes for cooking

Black bean and Quinoa Stuffed Bell Peppers

INGREDIENTS

- ❖ 4 bell peppers, cut in half, and seeds taken out
- ❖ One cup of black beans, one cup of cooked quinoa, and one cup of corn kernels
- ❖ one cup of tomatoes, chopped
- ❖ One teaspoon of cumin
- ❖ One tsp of chili powder
- ❖ To taste, add salt and pepper.
- ❖ To garnish, use fresh cilantro.

PREPARATION

- ❖ Turn the oven on to 375°F, or 190°C.
- ❖ The cooked quinoa, black beans, corn kernels, chopped tomatoes, cumin, chili powder, salt, and pepper should all be combined in a big bowl.
- ❖ Place the black bean and quinoa mixture into each half of a bell pepper.
- ❖ Pack the bell peppers and place them in a baking dish, covering them with foil.
- ❖ Bake the peppers for 25 to 30 minutes, or until they are soft.
- ❖ Take off the foil and continue baking for five more minutes to gently brown the tops.
- ❖ Before serving, garnish with fresh cilantro.

Nutrition Information

- ➢ Serving Size: Two half of pepper
- ➢ 280 calories
- ➢ 12g of protein
- ➢ 50g of carbohydrates
- ➢ 3g of fat
- ➢ 10g of fiber
- ➢ 15 minutes for preparation
- ➢ 35 minutes for cooking

Stir-fried Tofu with a Variety of Vegetables

INGREDIENTS

- One block of pressed and diced extra-firm tofu
- Two cups of mixed veggies, including snap peas, carrots, bell peppers, and broccoli
- three tsp of soy sauce
- Two tsp of hoisin sauce.
- One tablespoon of sesame oil
- two minced garlic cloves
- one tsp finely chopped ginger
- Prepared quinoa or brown rice for serving

PREPARATION

- In a large skillet or wok, heat the sesame oil over medium-high heat.
- Add the ginger and garlic, minced, and sauté until aromatic.
- When the cubed tofu is golden brown on both sides, add it to the skillet.
- Add the mixed veggies and stir until they become crisp-tender.
- Combine the hoisin sauce and soy sauce in a small bowl. Drizzle over the veggies and tofu.
- Cook for a further two to three minutes, stirring often.
- Serve cooked quinoa or brown rice with tofu stir-fry.

Nutrition Information

- One dish is served (either with rice or quinoa).
- 350 calories
- 20g of protein
- 40g of carbohydrates
- 15g of fat
- 8g of fiber
- 15 minutes for preparation
- 15 minutes is the cooking time.

Shepherd's Pie with Lentil and Mushrooms

INGREDIENTS

- two cups of boiled lentils
- One chopped onion
- two minced garlic cloves
- Two cups of chopped mushrooms
- One cup of veggie broth and one spoonful of tomato paste
- One teaspoon of thyme
- mashed potatoes (four to five potatoes are used)
- To taste, add salt and pepper.

PREPARATION

- Turn the oven on to 375°F, or 190°C.
- Diced onion and minced garlic should be cooked in a big pan until they are tender.
- Sliced mushrooms should be added and cooked until their moisture is released.
- Add the tomato paste, cooked lentils, vegetable broth, and thyme and stir. Simmer for ten minutes.
- To taste, add salt and pepper for seasoning.
- Spoon the mixture of lentils and mushrooms onto a baking dish.
- Mashed potatoes should be evenly spread over the top to thoroughly encase the contents.
- Bake the mashed potatoes for 25 to 30 minutes, or until they are golden brown.
- Before serving, let it cool for a few minutes.

Nutrition Information

- One slice is served.
- 280 calories
- 15g of protein
- 50g of carbohydrates
- 3g of fat
- 12g of fiber
- Twenty minutes for preparation
- 40 minutes for cooking

Tempeh-Vegan Chili

INGREDIENTS

- One container of crushed tempeh
- One sliced onion, two minced garlic cloves, one chopped bell pepper, one can (15 oz) of kidney beans that have been drained and washed
- One can (15 oz) of rinsed and drained black beans
- One (15-oz) can of chopped tomatoes
- Two cups of veggie broth and two tbsp of chili powder
- One teaspoon of cumin
- To taste, add salt and pepper.
- Cuts of avocado and fresh cilantro as garnish

PREPARATION

- Diced onion and minced garlic should be cooked till tender in a big saucepan.
- Cook the crumbled tempeh in the saucepan until it starts to color slightly.
- Add the diced tomatoes, kidney, black, and bell peppers; stir in the cumin, chili powder, and vegetable broth.
- Simmer the chili for twenty to twenty-five minutes, stirring from time to time.
- To taste, add salt and pepper for seasoning.
- Serve hot vegan chili with fresh cilantro and avocado slices as garnish.

Nutrition Information

- Serving size: one dish
- 320 calories
- 20g of protein
- 45g of carbohydrates
- 10g of fat
- 15g of fiber
- 15 minutes for preparation
- 25 minutes for cooking

Vegetarian Bolognese

INGREDIENTS

- Eight-ounce whole-wheat spaghetti
- One chopped onion
- two minced garlic cloves
- One grated carrot and one grated zucchini
- one cup of lentils, cooked
- One can (15 oz) chopped tomatoes
- TWO TABLEspoONS tomato paste
- One tsp of dehydrated oregano
- One tsp of dried basil
- To taste, add salt and pepper.
- For garnish, use fresh basil leaves.

PREPARATION

- Follow the cooking directions on the box for whole wheat spaghetti. After draining, put away.
- Diced onion and minced garlic should be cooked until aromatic in a big pan.
- Cook the zucchini and shredded carrot in the pan until they are tender.
- Add the dried oregano and dry basil, chopped tomatoes, cooked lentils, and tomato paste.
- Simmer the sauce for ten to fifteen minutes, or until the flavors combine.
- To taste, add salt and pepper for seasoning.
- Top cooked whole wheat spaghetti with vegan spaghetti bolognese and sprinkle with fresh basil.

Nutrition Information

- One dish is served.
- 350 calories
- 15g of protein
- 60g of carbohydrates
- 5g of fat
- 12g of fiber
- Ten minutes for preparation
- 20 minutes for cooking

Jackfruit and BBQ Vegan Sandwiches

INGREDIENTS

- Two 20-oz cans of young green jackfruit in brine that have been drained and shred
- One chopped onion
- two minced garlic cloves
- One cup of sauce for barbeques
- Four buns made with whole wheat
- Coleslaw as a garnish, if desired

PREPARATION

- Diced onion and minced garlic should be cooked in a big pan until they are tender.
- Cook the jackfruit shreds in the skillet until they are well heated.
- After adding the barbecue sauce, thoroughly mix it into the jackfruit.
- Simmer the jackfruit in the sauce for ten to fifteen minutes, or until the flavors combine.
- Whole wheat burger buns should be softly browned after toasting.
- Place a vegan BBQ jackfruit spoonful on the underside of every bun.
- If desired, place coleslaw on top before covering with the upper portion of the bread.
- Warm up vegan barbecued jackfruit sandwiches.

Nutrition Information

- One sandwich per serving size
- 320 calories
- 10g of protein
- 60g of carbohydrates
- 5g of fat
- 8g of fiber
- Ten minutes for preparation
- 20 minutes for cooking

Veggie and Bean Vegan Tacos

INGREDIENTS

- One can (15 oz) of rinsed and drained black beans
- One chopped onion, two minced garlic cloves, and one diced bell pepper
- One cup of kernel corn
- One teaspoon of cumin
- One tsp of chili powder
- To taste, add salt and pepper.
- Tacos made with corn
- Slices of avocado with salsa as garnish

PREPARATION

- Diced onion and minced garlic should be cooked until aromatic in a big pan.
- Cook the corn kernels and chopped bell pepper in the pan until they are soft.
- Add the chili powder, cumin, black beans, salt, and pepper and stir.
- Cook until the bean and vegetable mixture is cooked through, about 5 to 7 minutes.
- Corn tortillas may be reheated in a microwave or dry skillet.
- Spoon combination of beans and vegetables onto each tortilla.
- Add salsa and avocado slices on top.
- Hot bean and vegetable tacos made without dairy.

Nutrition Information

- Quantity served: two tacos
- 300 calories
- 12g of protein
- 50g of carbohydrates
- 5g of fat
- 10g of fiber
- Ten minutes for preparation
- 15 minutes is the cooking time.

Vegetarian Pesto Parmesan

INGREDIENTS

- ❖ One big eggplant cut into rounds
- ❖ one cup of breadcrumbs
- ❖ One cup of marinara sauce
- ❖ One cup of shredded vegan mozzarella cheese
- ❖ 1/4 cup of nutritional yeast
- ❖ For garnish, use fresh basil leaves.
- ❖ Using olive oil to brush

PREPARATION

- ❖ Turn the oven on to 375°F, or 190°C.
- ❖ Slices of eggplant are brushed with olive oil and then dipped in bread crumbs.
- ❖ Arrange the breaded eggplant slices onto a parchment paper-lined baking sheet.
- ❖ Bake the eggplant slices for 20 to 25 minutes, or until they are soft and golden brown.
- ❖ Line a baking dish's bottom with marinara sauce.
- ❖ Arrange the pieces of roasted eggplant in the baking dish.
- ❖ Drizzle the eggplant slices with nutritional yeast and vegan mozzarella cheese.
- ❖ For a further 10 to 15 minutes, or until the cheese is melted and bubbling, bake the vegan eggplant parmesan.
- ❖ Before serving, garnish with fresh basil leaves.

Nutrition Information

- ➢ One dish is served.
- ➢ 320 calories
- ➢ 15g of protein
- ➢ 40g of carbohydrates
- ➢ 10g of fat
- ➢ 8g of fiber
- ➢ 15 minutes for preparation
- ➢ 40 minutes for cooking

Risotto with vegan mushrooms

INGREDIENTS

- ❖ One cup Arborio rice
- ❖ One chopped onion
- ❖ two minced garlic cloves
- ❖ Two cups of chopped mushrooms
- ❖ Four cups veggie broth and one-half cup of optional white wine
- ❖ 1/4 cup of nutritional yeast
- ❖ Two tsp vegan butter
- ❖ To taste, add salt and pepper.
- ❖ As a garnish, use fresh parsley.

PREPARATION

- ❖ Diced onion and minced garlic should be cooked in a big pot until they are tender.
- ❖ Sliced mushrooms should be added to the pot and cooked until their moisture is released.
- ❖ Cook for a further minute after adding the Arborio rice.
- ❖ If using white wine, add it now and boil until it is absorbed.
- ❖ Stirring continuously, gradually add the vegetable broth to the pot until the rice is cooked and creamy.
- ❖ Add vegan butter and nutritional yeast, then taste and adjust with salt and pepper.
- ❖ Risotto should be taken off the heat and left for a few minutes to thicken.
- ❖ Before serving, garnish with fresh parsley.

Nutrition Information

- ➢ Serving size: one dish
- ➢ 350 calories
- ➢ 10g of protein
- ➢ 60g of carbohydrates
- ➢ 5g of fat
- ➢ 8g of fiber
- ➢ Ten minutes for preparation
- ➢ 30 minutes for cooking

Chapter 5

SNACKS AND TREATS FOR FUELING WORKOUTS

Balls of High-Protein Energy

INGREDIENTS

- ❖ One cup of rolled oats
- ❖ half a cup of almond butter
- ❖ One-fourth cup maple syrup
- ❖ Two tsp of chia seeds
- ❖ Two tsp vegan protein powder
- ❖ Optional: 1/4 cup dark chocolate chips

PREPARATION

- ❖ Mix all ingredients together in a large mixing basin until well combined.
- ❖ Using your hands, roll the mixture into bite-sized balls.
- ❖ To make the energy balls firmer, place them on a baking sheet covered with parchment paper and chill for at least half an hour.
- ❖ After cooling down, keep the energy balls in the fridge for up to a week by placing them in an airtight container.

Nutrition Information

- ➢ Serving Size: One energy ball
- ➢ 120 calories
- ➢ 5g of protein
- ➢ 12g of carbohydrates
- ➢ 6g of fat
- ➢ 2g of fiber
- ➢ Ten minutes for preparation

- ➢ 30 minutes is the chill time.

Trail Mix Packed with Protein

INGREDIENTS

- ❖ One cup of mixed nuts (walnuts, cashews, and almonds)
- ❖ half a cup of pumpkin seeds
- ❖ Dried cranberries, half a cup
- ❖ One-fourth cup of dark chocolate chips
- ❖ 1/4 cup of coconut flakes

PREPARATION

- ❖ Combine all ingredients in a big bowl and stir until well combined.
- ❖ Place the trail mix in tiny, resealable bags or containers and divide it into individual portions.

Nutrition Information

- ➢ 1/4 cup is the serving size.
- ➢ 200 calories
- ➢ 7g of protein
- ➢ 15g of carbohydrates
- ➢ 14g of fat
- ➢ 3g of fiber
- ➢ Five minutes for preparation
One hour is the chill time

Bites of Chickpea Cookie Dough

INGREDIENTS

- ❖ One can of washed and drained chickpeas
- ❖ one-fourth cup almond butter
- ❖ One-fourth cup maple syrup
- ❖ One tsp vanilla essence
- ❖ One-fourth cup of dark chocolate chips

PREPARATION

- ❖ Puree the chickpeas, almond butter, maple syrup, and vanilla essence in a food processor until creamy.
- ❖ Add chocolate chunks and stir.
- ❖ Form the dough into little balls and place them in the refrigerator to solidify.

Nutrition Information

- ➤ Serving Size: One Bite
- ➤ 70 calories
- ➤ 3g of protein
- ➤ 9g of carbohydrates
- ➤ 3g of fat
- ➤ 2g of fiber
- ➤ Ten minutes for preparation
- ➤ 30 minutes is the chill time.

Plant-Based Protein Pancakes

INGREDIENTS

- ❖ One cup of flour made from whole wheat
- ❖ One scoop of plant-based protein powder
- ❖ One-third tsp baking powder
- ❖ One spoonful of flaxseed meal
- ❖ One cup almond milk
- ❖ One spoonful of maple syrup
- ❖ One tsp vanilla essence

PREPARATION

- ❖ Mix the flour, baking powder, protein powder, and flaxseed in a big bowl.
- ❖ Add the vanilla extract, maple syrup, and almond milk and stir until smooth.
- ❖ Pour batter onto a nonstick skillet set over medium heat to make pancakes.
- ❖ Cook until surface bubbles appear, then turn and continue cooking until golden brown.
- ❖ Top with your preferred ingredients, such as nut butter, sliced bananas, or berries.

Nutrition Information

- ➤ Two pancakes are served.
- ➤ 250 calories
- ➤ 15g of protein
- ➤ 35g of carbohydrates
- ➤ 5g of fat
- ➤ 6g of fiber
- ➤ Ten minutes for preparation
- ➤ Ten minutes to cook

Avocado Pudding with Chocolate and Protein

INGREDIENTS

- ❖ Two ripe avocados
- ❖ One-fourth cup cocoa powder
- ❖ One-fourth cup maple syrup
- ❖ One scoop of plant-based chocolate protein powder
- ❖ One tsp vanilla essence
- ❖ A dash of salt

PREPARATION

- ❖ Process avocados in a food processor until smooth.
- ❖ Blend in protein powder, salt, vanilla extract, protein powder, and cocoa powder until smooth.
- ❖ Let it cool for a minimum of half an hour before serving.

Nutrition Information

- ➢ Portion Size: half a cup
- ➢ 200 calories
- ➢ 8g of protein
- ➢ 20g of carbohydrates
- ➢ 12g of fat
- ➢ 6g of fiber
- ➢ Ten minutes for preparation
- ➢ 30 minutes is the chill time.

Quinoa Energy Bars

INGREDIENTS

- ❖ One cup of cooked quinoa
- ❖ Half a cup of rolled oats
- ❖ one-fourth cup almond butter
- ❖ One-fourth cup maple syrup
- ❖ 1/4 cup of finely chopped nuts, such walnuts or almonds
- ❖ 1/4 cup of dried fruit, preferably chopped dates or raisins

PREPARATION

- ❖ Almond butter, maple syrup, cooked quinoa, and oats should all be well mixed together in a big bowl.
- ❖ Add the dried fruit and chopped nuts and stir.
- ❖ After pressing the mixture into a baking dish that has been lined, chill it for at least an hour.
- ❖ Once solid, slice into bars and keep chilled.

Nutrition Information

- ➢ One bar is served.
- ➢ 180 calories
- ➢ 6g of protein
- ➢ 25g of carbohydrates
- ➢ 7g of fat
- ➢ 4g of fiber
- ➢ Ten minutes for preparation
- ➢ One hour is the chill time.

Muffins with Sweet Potato Protein

INGREDIENTS

* Two cups of sweet potatoes, mashed
* one-fourth cup almond butter
* One-fourth cup maple syrup
* one-fourth cup almond milk
* One tsp vanilla essence and one cup of whole wheat flour.
* One scoop of plant-based protein powder
* One tsp baking powder
* half a teaspoon of cinnamon
* A dash of salt

PREPARATION

* Grease a muffin tray with cooking spray and preheat the oven to 350°F (175°C).
* Mashed sweet potatoes, almond butter, maple syrup, almond milk, and vanilla extract should all be combined smoothly in a big dish.
* Mix the flour, baking powder, cinnamon, protein powder, and salt in a another basin.
* Stirring until just blended, gradually add the dry ingredients to the wet ones.
* When a toothpick inserted into the middle comes out clean, bake the muffins for 20 to 25 minutes, dividing the batter equally among the cups.
* Muffins should cool before being served.

Nutrition Information

* One muffin per serving
* 150 calories
* 6g of protein
* 25g of carbohydrates
* 4g of fat
* 3g of fiber
* 15 minutes for preparation
* Cooking Time: 20 to 25 minutes

Plant-Based Protein Bars

INGREDIENTS

* One cup of rolled oats
* Half a cup of vegan protein powder
* one-fourth cup almond butter
* One-fourth cup maple syrup
* one-fourth cup almond milk
* 1/4 cup of finely chopped nuts, such cashews or almonds
* 1/4 cup of dried fruit, such apricots or cranberries

PREPARATION

* Almond butter, maple syrup, almond milk, protein powder, and oats should all be well mixed together in a big bowl.
* Add the dried fruit and chopped nuts and stir.
* After pressing the mixture into a baking dish that has been lined, chill it for at least an hour.
* Once solid, slice into bars and keep chilled.

Nutrition Information

* One bar is served.
* 200 calories; 10g of protein
* 20g of carbohydrates
* 8g of fat
* 3g of fiber
* Ten minutes for preparation
* One hour is the chill time.

Peanut Butter and Banana Protein Smoothie

INGREDIENTS

- ❖ One ripe banana
- ❖ One scoop of vegan protein powder (chocolate or vanilla)
- ❖ One spoonful of peanut butter
- ❖ One cup almond milk
- ❖ Scoop of ice cubes

PREPARATION

- ❖ Banana, protein powder, peanut butter, almond milk, and ice cubes should all be combined in a blender.
- ❖ Blend till creamy and smooth.
- ❖ Pour into a glass and start sipping right away.

Nutrition Information

- ➢ One smoothie is served per serving.
- ➢ 300 calories
- ➢ 20g of protein
- ➢ 30g of carbohydrates
- ➢ 10g of fat
- ➢ 5g of fiber
- ➢ Five minutes for preparation

Smoothie with Berries Blast

INGREDIENTS

- ❖ One cup of frozen mixed berries
- ❖ One ripe banana
- ❖ one cup of spinach
- ❖ One spoonful of chia seeds
- ❖ One cup almond milk

PREPARATION

- ❖ In blender, combine all ingredients.
- ❖ Blend till creamy and smooth.
- ❖ Pour into a glass and start sipping right away.

Nutrition Information

- ➢ 250 calories
- ➢ 7g of protein
- ➢ 45g of carbohydrates
- ➢ 6g of fat
- ➢ 12g of fiber
- ➢ Five minutes for preparation
- ➢ Time Spent Cooking: 0 minutes

Chapter 6

BONUS RECIPES FOR PERFORMANCE ENHANCEMENT

Pre-Workout Smoothies and Snacks

Banana and Peanut Butter Protein Smoothie

INGREDIENTS

- Two fully ripe bananas
- Two tsp of peanut butter
- One scoop of plant-based protein powder
- One cup almond milk
- Cubes of ice (optional)

PREPARATION

- After peeling, put the bananas in a blender.
- Stir in almond milk, peanut butter, protein powder, and ice cubes (if using).
- Blend till creamy and smooth.
- After pouring into a glass, savor!

Nutrition Information

- 380 calories
- 25g of protein
- 35g of carbohydrates
- 15g of fat
- 8g of fiber
- Five minutes for preparation
- Time Spent Cooking: 0 minutes

The Green Power Smoothie

INGREDIENTS

- One cup of kale
- half a cucumber, sliced and peeled
- One green apple, peeled and diced
- One tablespoon of freshly peeled and sliced ginger; one tablespoon of lemon juice
- One cup of coconut water

PREPARATION

- Put everything into a blender.
- Blend until thoroughly integrated and smooth.
- Taste and add extra apple or lemon juice if needed to balance the sweetness.
- Transfer into a glass and serve right away.

Nutrition Information

- 150 calories
- 3g of protein
- 35g of carbohydrates
- Fat: 1 gram
- Fiber: nine grams
- Five minutes for preparation
- Time Spent Cooking: 0 minutes

Nut-rich Chocolate Energy Balls

INGREDIENTS

- ❖ One cup of rolled oats
- ❖ half a cup of almond butter
- ❖ One-fourth cup maple syrup
- ❖ Two tsp of cocoa powder
- ❖ 1/4 cup of almonds, chopped
- ❖ A dash of salt

PREPARATION

- ❖ Rolling oats, almond butter, maple syrup, chocolate powder, sliced nuts, and salt should all be well mixed together in a big basin.
- ❖ With your hands, roll the mixture into little balls.
- ❖ Arrange the energy balls on a parchment paper-lined baking sheet.
- ❖ Before serving, let the food cool for at least half an hour in the refrigerator.

Nutrition Information

- ➤ 90 calories a ball.
- ➤ 3g of protein
- ➤ 8g of carbohydrates
- ➤ 5g of fat
- ➤ 2g of fiber
- ➤ Ten minutes for preparation
- ➤ Time Spent Cooking: 0 minutes

Avocado and Chickpea Toast

INGREDIENTS

- ❖ One mature avocado
- ❖ One can of washed and drained chickpeas
- ❖ One tablespoon of lemon juice
- ❖ one-fourth teaspoon powdered garlic
- ❖ To taste, add salt and pepper.
- ❖ Four toasted whole grain pieces of bread

PREPARATION

- ❖ Mash the avocado until it's smooth in a bowl.
- ❖ To the bowl, add the chickpeas, lemon juice, garlic powder, salt, and pepper.
- ❖ Blend everything until fully mixed, adding just enough chunks of chickpeas for texture.
- ❖ Toast the bread pieces and spread the avocado-chickpea mixture on them.
- ❖ Enjoy and serve right now!

Nutrition Information

- ➤ 250 calories for two slices of food.
- ➤ 10g of protein
- ➤ 35g of carbohydrates
- ➤ 8g of fat
- ➤ 12g of fiber
- ➤ Ten minutes for preparation
- ➤ Five minutes to cook

Chocolate Peanut Butter Protein Shake

INGREDIENTS

❖ One ripe banana
❖ Two tsp natural peanut butter
❖ One scoop of plant-based chocolate protein powder
❖ 1 cup almond milk without sugar
❖ One spoonful of powdered cacao
❖ Cubes of ice (optional)

PREPARATION

❖ Fill a blender with all the ingredients.
❖ Blend till creamy and smooth.
❖ To get a cooler consistency, feel free to add ice cubes and mix once more.
❖ Pour into a glass and start sipping right away.

Nutrition Information

➤ 380 calories
➤ 25g of protein
➤ 32g of carbohydrates
➤ 18g of fat
➤ 7g of fiber
➤ Five minutes for preparation
➤ Time Spent Cooking: 0 minutes

Green Power Smoothie

INGREDIENTS

❖ one cup of raw spinach
❖ Half a ripe avocado
❖ Half a cup of frozen pineapple chunks
❖ One serving of vegan vanilla protein powder
❖ One spoonful of chia seeds
❖ One cup of coconut water

PREPARATION

❖ Put everything into a blender.
❖ Blend till creamy and smooth.
❖ If necessary, adjust the consistency by adding more coconut water.
❖ Transfer into a glass and serve right away.

Nutrition Information

➤ 320 calories
➤ 20g of protein
➤ 30g of carbohydrates
➤ 15g of fat
➤ 10g of fiber
➤ Five minutes for preparation
➤ Time Spent Cooking: 0 minutes

Turmeric Mango Recovery Shake

INGREDIENTS

- One cup of frozen mango chunks
- One ripe banana
- half a teaspoon of turmeric powder
- One serving of vegan vanilla protein powder
- One-third tsp flaxseed meal
- One cup of coconut milk without sugar

PREPARATION

- Fill a blender with all the ingredients.
- Blend till creamy and smooth.
- If desired, adjust sweetness by adding more banana.
- Transfer into a glass and serve right away.

Nutrition Information

- 310 calories
- 20g of protein
- 35g of carbohydrates
- 10g of fat
- 8g of fiber
- Five minutes for preparation
- Time Spent Cooking: 0 minutes

Coffee Cacao Protein Shake

INGREDIENTS

- One cup of cooled brewed coffee
- Half a cup of unflavored almond milk
- One scoop of plant-based chocolate protein powder
- One spoonful of nibs de cacao
- One tablespoon of maple syrup, if desired
- Cubes of ice (optional)

PREPARATION

- In blender, combine all ingredients.
- Process until foamy and smooth.
- If desired, use maple syrup to modify sweetness based on taste.
- To get a cooler consistency, add the ice cubes and combine once more.
- Pour into a glass and start sipping right away.

Nutrition Information

- 250 calories
- 20g of protein
- 20g of carbohydrates
- 10g of fat
- 5g of fiber
- Five minutes for preparation
- Time Spent Cooking: 0 minutes

Chickpea Protein Bars

INGREDIENTS

- two cups of boiled lentils
- half a cup of almond butter
- One-fourth cup maple syrup
- 1/4 cup of powdered protein (hemp or pea protein)
- One-fourth cup rolled oats
- 1/4 cup of finely chopped nuts, such walnuts or almonds
- 1/4 cup of dried fruit, preferably chopped dates or raisins
- One tsp vanilla essence
- A dash of salt

PREPARATION

- Adjust the oven temperature to 350°F (175°C) and place parchment paper in a baking dish.
- Chickpeas, almond butter, maple syrup, protein powder, oats, almonds, dried fruit, vanilla extract, and salt should all be combined in a food processor. Process till smooth.
- Spread the mixture evenly in the baking dish that has been prepared.
- Bake for twenty to twenty-five minutes, or until the sides are browned.
- Take out of the oven and let it cool fully before slicing it into bars.
- For up to a week, keep in the refrigerator in an airtight container.

Nutrition Information

- One bar is served.
- 200 calories; 10g of protein
- 20g of carbohydrates
- 8g of fat
- 5g of fiber
- Ten minutes for preparation
- Cooking Time: 20 to 25 minutes

Soy Protein Shake

INGREDIENTS

- One cup of unflavored soy milk
- One ripe banana
- One spoonful of peanut butter
- One scoop of protein powder made from soy
- half a teaspoon of cinnamon
- Scoop of ice cubes

PREPARATION

- Blend together the ice cubes, banana, peanut butter, soy protein powder, cinnamon, and soy milk in a blender.
- Blend till creamy and smooth.
- Pour into a glass and start sipping right away.

Nutrition Information

- One shake per serving
- 300 calories
- 25g of protein
- 30g of carbohydrates
- 10g of fat
- 5g of fiber
- Five minutes for preparation
- Time Spent Cooking: 0 minutes

Protein Balls Made with Hemp

INGREDIENTS

- ❖ One cup of rolled oats
- ❖ Hemp protein powder, half a cup
- ❖ one-fourth cup almond butter
- ❖ One-fourth cup maple syrup
- ❖ 1/4 cup of coconut, shredded
- ❖ One tsp vanilla essence
- ❖ A dash of salt

PREPARATION

- ❖ Rolling oats, hemp protein powder, almond butter, maple syrup, shredded coconut, vanilla essence, and salt should all be combined in a big bowl.
- ❖ Blend until well blended.
- ❖ Make little balls out of the mixture using your hands.
- ❖ To firm up the balls, place them on a baking sheet covered with parchment paper and chill for at least half an hour.
- ❖ For up to a week, keep in the refrigerator in an airtight container.

Nutrition Information

- ➢ Serving size: one ball
- ➢ 100 calories
- ➢ 5g of protein
- ➢ 10g of carbohydrates
- ➢ 5g of fat
- ➢ 2g of fiber
- ➢ Ten minutes for preparation
- ➢ Time Spent Cooking: 0 minutes

Pumpkin Seed Protein Bars

INGREDIENTS

- ❖ one cup of seeds from pumpkins
- ❖ Dried cranberries, half a cup
- ❖ 1/4 cup protein powder, such as that found in pumpkin seeds or peas.
- ❖ one-fourth cup almond butter
- ❖ One-fourth cup maple syrup
- ❖ One tsp of cinnamon
- ❖ A dash of salt

PREPARATION

- ❖ Pumpkin seeds, protein powder, almond butter, maple syrup, cinnamon, salt, and dried cranberries should all be combined in a food processor.
- ❖ Pulse just until the mixture forms a sticky dough and comes together.
- ❖ Smooth the top after pressing the dough onto a baking dish that has been lined.
- ❖ To set, refrigerate for a minimum of one hour.
- ❖ Cut into bars and refrigerate for up to a week in an airtight container.

Nutrition Information

- ➢ One bar is served.
- ➢ 150 calories; 8g of protein
- ➢ 15g of carbohydrates
- ➢ 7g of fat
- ➢ 3g of fiber
- ➢ Ten minutes for preparation
- ➢ Time Spent Cooking: 0 minutes

INGREDIENTS:

1. One cup of cooked quinoa
2. Half a cup of cooked or canned black beans, rinsed and drained
3. Half a cup of cubed tofu and half a cup of chopped veggies (such tomatoes, cucumbers, and bell peppers)
4. Twice as much tahini
5. One tablespoon of lemon juice
6. One spoonful of nutritious yeast
7. To taste, add salt and pepper.

INSTRUCTIONS:

1. The cooked quinoa, chopped veggies, black beans, and tofu should all be combined in a dish.
2. To prepare the dressing, combine the tahini, nutritional yeast, lemon juice, salt, and pepper in a separate small bowl.
3. After adding the dressing to the quinoa mixture, toss to ensure uniform coating.
4. Spoon the mixture into bowls and serve right away, or refrigerate for up to three days in an airtight container.

Nutrition per Serving:

- ❖ One bowl is the serving size.
- ❖ 300 calories
- ❖ 15g of protein
- ❖ 30g of carbohydrates
- ❖ 12g of fat
- ❖ 8g of fiber
- ❖ 15 minutes for preparation
- ❖ Cooking time for tofu and quinoa is 15 minutes.

Conclusion

As we come to the end of our Vegan Bodybuilding Cookbook, I can't help but think back on the amazing adventure we've been on together. Every dish has been a labor of love and a tribute to the transformational power of plant-based nutrition, from the tempting scent of sizzling stir-fries to the gratifying crunch of protein-packed energy balls.

We've examined the relationship between veganism and bodybuilding in these pages, going into the science of muscle development, the art of meal preparation, and the endless possibilities of plant-powered performance. However, there is a deeper reality that goes beyond dietary advice and nutritional insights. This truth touches on the core of what it is to be human.

Vegan bodybuilding is a deep expression of compassion, perseverance, and connection for me—it's about more than simply growing a physique or reaching personal objectives. It's about appreciating our bodies' amazing capacities and upholding the sacredness of all life on Earth. It's about creating a route to health that feeds our spirit as well as our body.

I want to express my sincere appreciation to all of the readers and would-be vegan bodybuilders who have joined me on this trip. Your passion, inquisitiveness, and commitment have propelled this project forward and motivated me to push the limits of culinary and nutritional innovation.

Remind yourself that you are much more competent than you ever would have thought as you go on your journey to vegan bodybuilding perfection. Have faith in your body's knowledge, your mind's ability, and your spirit's tenacity. Accept every obstacle as a chance for personal development, every disappointment as a reminder to persevere, and every accomplishment as a testament to your limitless potential.

So let's preserve the knowledge gained, the recipes enjoyed, and the relationships developed while we say goodbye to these pages. On this incredible adventure we call life, let's continue to feed our interests, take care of our bodies, and encourage one another.